The Tubby Theory From Topeka

The Tubby Theory From Topeka

An Analysis of a Lipidologist's Medical
Practice in Topeka, Kansas

Brian S. Edwards, MD, and Luke M. Edwards

To order additional copies of this book, contact:
Xlibris Corporation
1-888-795-4274
www.Xlibris.com
Orders@Xlibris.com
72521

CONTENTS

Regression of Carotid Atheroma with CIMT

	right	left			LDL-P	HDL-P
6/1/07	0.639	0.743	Arteriovision TM	on statin and Endur-acin	1,008	38.9
7/29/08	0.50	0.58	Phillips IU 22 ultrasound	went off Endur-acin 1/1/09	534	31.9
11/19/09	0.52	0.54	Phillips IU 22 ultrasound		761	37.7
12-17-09	avg. mean 0.599 mm SonoCalc IMT			Weight 248 pounds		

These are my scores. The first score in 2007 is not statin naive. I had been on statins since my diabetes diagnosis in 1999.

I hope that in the future, high-risk patients will also be following their CIMT scores as a standard routine.

No radiation.
Cost is $100.
Semiautomated machine improves reliability.
Software read off 99% reliable reading on the third CIMT.

SonoCalc™ IMT Scan Report

Common Carotid Artery Intima-Media Thickness (IMT) V 3.4.0.5

EDWARDS, BRIAN

Date of Birth: 12-27-1951
Age at Exam: 57
Gender: M
Ethnic Origin: White or Other
Patient ID: 9907081
Exam. Date: 12-17-2009
Report Created: 12-17-2009

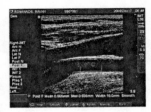

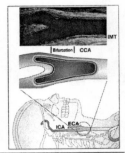

Average CCA Mean IMT:

Average of individual mean IMT measurements

0.599mm

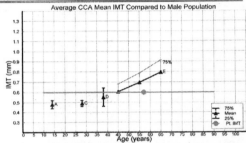

Average CCA Max Region IMT:

Average of individual 1mm Max Region measurements

0.741mm

Grossly Unremarkable

12/18/09

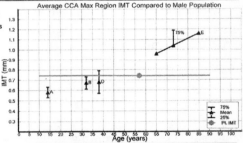

A Tonstad, S (1996) Arterioscler Thromb D Tonstad, S (1998) Eur J Clin Invest
B Urbina, E (2002) Am J Cardiol   E Aminbakhsh, A (1999) Clin Invest Med
C Oren, A (2003) Arch Intern Med.

See User Guide for complete references. All reference data is 10mm distal CCA
and is primarily from white populations with no coronary history. Consult your
Doctor for information on race differences.

SonoCalc™ IMT

SonoSite.

Your Doctor should interpret this IMT result in conjunction with your other risk factors. Medical decision making takes a
multitude of factors into account, and risk factor modification should be made in consultation with your Doctor .

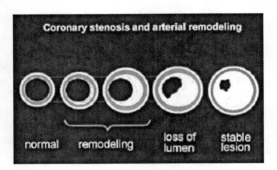

The Message of This Book

The Tubby theory is that we can prevent heart disease with simvastatin/ Endur-acin in America for less than $90 a year if we find the subclinical atherosclerosis early with CAC/CIMT.

The *Tubby Factor* = non-HDL cholesterol level = total cholesterol minus HDL-C = The *Tubby Factor* $_{TM}$

The *Tubby syndrome* = metabolic syndrome = waist >35" female/40" male, BP systolic >129, Glucose >99, HDL-C <50, TG > 149

Three or more of these factors qualifies as having the Tubby syndrome. This is what causes the inflammation of the plaque to make it unstable and rupture which may cause sudden death or stroke.

The Tubby Guidelines (Blood Test on Standard Lipid Panel)

Primary goal:
> The Tubby Factor goal = **< 80** (non-HDL cholesterol)

Secondary goals:
> HDL-C **> 50** or HDL-P **> 35**
> > Triglycerides **< 100**

The Tubby Plan

> Obtain CAC (calcium score) and CIMT (carotid intima-media thickness) to determine if there is plaque or atheroma.
> Obtain NMR LipoScience LipoProfile to determine the LDL-P (blood test).
> Combination Therapy
> > Simvastatin $10 for three months treatment

Endur-acin (niacin) 500 mg twice a day with meals, $70 for 1,000 tabs purchased on Internet

DHA/EPA more than 850 mg a day (Fish oil tablets over the counter are okay.)

Vitamin D3 2,000 IU a day in oil-based capsule.

The Tubby Lifestyle Change

Exercise: Start with eight-minute walks after meals and back exercise (arms around knees before getting out of bed).

Tubby diet: Eat every three hours exactly as outlined on Tubby diet sheets.

LDL-P (LDL particle number obtained by NMR LipoScience LipoProfile)—the measurement of the lipoprotein that carries the cholesterol

The LDL-P number is more predictive of outcome than LDL-C or the Tubby Factor (non-HDL cholesterol).

Medicare pays for this, but most private insurance companies do not. It costs about $100 and should be done at least once to make certain that there is not a discordance with the LDL-C or the Tubby Factor. The LDL-P goal is less than 750 for very high-risk patients.

The Paradigm Shift: Find subclinical atherosclerosis with a CAC and CIMT to stabilize vulnerable plaque from inflammation and rupture.

The cholesterol *content*
LDL-C
HDL-C

vs.

The number of *vehicles* carrying the cholesterol
LDL-P
HDL-P

The cholesterol found in the plasma is carried in the particles (vehicles). Some particles carry more cholesterol than others.

Measuring the cholesterol in the plasma (LDL-C) will not tell you how many particles are in the plasma (LDL-P).

The same is true with HDL-C and HDL-P.

The NMR (nuclear magnetic resonance) machine measures the number of particles.

APOB immunoassay is another way to measure the number of particles. Every atherogenic particle has one APOB on it.

The atherogenic particles include LDL-P, VLDL-P, IDL-P, chylomicrons, and lipoprotein (a) and remnants.

I use the NMR LipoScience LipoProfile because Medicare pays for it.

I use the old routine lipid panel only on patients with private insurance. The Tubby Factor is obtained without additional expense on the old lipid panel by the following calculation:

TOTAL CHOLESTEROL
-HDL-C
NON-HDL CHOLESTEROL
(TUBBY FACTOR)

< = less than

> = more than

CIMT (carotid intima-media thickness)—ultrasound of carotid arteries in the neck to measure thickness of the carotid wall. This is not paid for by insurance. This is not to be confused with duplex or triplex carotid ultrasound, which measures the flow of the blood and gives a calculation of the amount of blockage (stenosis) of the lumen of the carotid artery. This test is usually $600, and insurance often will pay for it. The duplex carotid ultrasound is also what Lifeline usually does for a reduced price in churches.

CAC (coronary artery calcium)—calcium score of the heart. Calcium score of 1.0 or greater means there is coronary plaque. Zero is normal, but in a young person, it may be a false negative, as the soft plaque has not been calcified yet. In a symptomatic patient (i.e., a patient with chest pain), it is more likely to be a false negative with a zero score; but in an asymptomatic patient, it signifies a very good prognosis for three years. This is a CT scan with radiation but no IV dye or isotope injection.

Non-HDL cholesterol (total cholesterol minus HDL-C or *Tubby Factor*)—This blood test has been an NCEP guideline goal after achieving LDL-C goal if triglycerides are more than 200. For people with private insurance, this is the best single test, better than the LDL-C. Don't bother with the LDL-C goal if your *Tubby Factor* is less than 80.

LDL-P (LDL particle number)—This is the most predictive of the lipids. It is a blood test that is sent to North Carolina to be done with an NMR machine. The goal is less than 750 for very high-risk patients and less than 1,000 for high-risk patients. Medicare pays for this. I usually have a private insurance patient pay $100 out of pocket once a year to determine if there is LDL-C discordance with LDL-P. This is very common in patients with the *Tubby syndrome* (metabolic syndrome).

HDL-C (high-density lipoprotein cholesterol or the good cholesterol)—Very low levels and very high levels are probably not good. HDL-C less than 40 is considered a major risk factor. HDL-C more than 60 is considered to lower risk in the Framingham score. ADA guidelines call for HDL-C more than 50. Thus the *Tubby guidelines* shoots for an HDL-C more than 50. This does not give the critical information about the *functionality* of the HDL-P. Even if the HDL-P is more than 35, we have no idea about the functionality of the HDL. It could be pro-inflammatory. In other words, it could be a bad lipid.

LDL-C (low-density lipoprotein cholesterol)—the evidence-based gold standard, the lower the LDL-C the better the outcome. No question about it. So why is the Tubby Factor and the LDL-P a better test? In Tubby syndrome (metabolic syndrome) patients, the LDL-C is low because of the high triglycerides. There is a high VLDL-P and other particles not being picked up by the LDL-C. This is true of diabetics as well.

NCEP Definitions of Lipid Ranges

Optimal: associated with very low risk of atherosclerosis (LDL-P < 1,000 or LDL-C < 100)

Above optimal: *atherosclerosis occurs at this level (LDL-P 1,000-1,299 or LDL-C >100)*

Borderline high: atherosclerosis occurs at a significant rate (LDL-P 1,300-1,599)

High and very high: atherosclerosis proceeds at a markedly accelerated rate (LDL-P > 1,600)

Statins: These drugs decrease cholesterol production in the liver and increase the LDL receptors in the liver, which takes LDL-Ps out of the blood.

Crestor (rosuvastatin): Strongest statin. Very safe especially in terms of liver safety. JUPITER trial.

Lipitor (atorvastatin): Good for renal insufficient patients. Very safe. Prove-it trial. TNT

Zocor (simvastatin): The star statin from seminal drug trials such as HPS and 4S. Now available as generic for $10 for three months. Avoid using the 80 mg dose.

Pravachol (pravastatin): good for HIV patients

Leschol XL 80 mg (fluvastatin): The go-to drug in patients who can't tolerate statins. No reported cases of rhabdomyolysis.

Endur-acin: sustained-release niacin. At 1,000 mg, it is safe in terms of raising glucose or affecting the liver. This brand seems to have very little flushing.

Flush-free niacin: No effect on lipid profile. Not nicotinic acid.

Niaspan: Extended-release nicotinic acid. The brand name of niacin that is safer for the liver in high doses. This is an option if a physician does not want to use Zetia and would rather use 2,000 mg of niacin to lower LDL-C. The HDL-C does not increase much more with doses above 1,000 mg. Good luck trying to get the patient to take it.

Immediate-release niacin: This is the safest niacin in terms of liver toxicity, but it is also the most difficult to take due to flushing.

Zetia: Blocks absorption of cholesterol. This is often the drug needed to get to lipid goal. The body tends to absorb more cholesterol to compensate for the decrease production of cholesterol caused by a statin. SEAS trial had a positive secondary end point to reduce ischemic events. SANDS trial did reduce atheroma in CIMT study.

Trilipex: good drug to lower TG and raise small-size HDL-P. The only drug with FDA indication to use with a statin. Good add-on drug for diabetics. Beware of Lopid (gemfibrozil) from this group.

Welchol: bile-acid-binding resin. Six pills a day are difficult to take due to some constipation. Important tip: just two a day with another lipid-lowering drug can have good results. The CCPT trial used cholestyramine which settled the cholesterol theory controversy. Cholestyramine is a similar drug. This class of drugs is not absorbed. This drug may raise TG, so do not use if TGs are elevated.

The Complex World of HDL

NMR LipoScience	Berkeley	Boston HeartLab
H1 or H2 HDL3	alpha 3 or 4	Small HDL
H4 or H5 HDL2	alpha 2 or 1	More mature larger HDL
prebeta HDL: the immature form of HDL		

CAD: coronary artery disease

CHD: cerebrovascular heart disease

CVD: cardiovascular heart disease

IVUS: Intravascular ultrasound (a small doppler at the end of an angiocatheter looks at the artery from the inside out; it shows all the plaque). The plaque in the lumen and the atheroma in the wall of the artery

Coronary angiogram: "lumenogram," the dye inserted through a catheter to the coronary arteries shows if there is stenosis (blockage) in the artery. It does not show the atheroma in the wall of the artery.

APOB: apolipoprotein B is present on all the atherogenic particles, including LDL-P, IDL-P, VLDL-P, chylomicrons, and apo(a).

NCEP: National Cholesterol Education Program

ATP (Adult Treatment Panel): This is where the lipid guidelines from the NCEP come from. We are awaiting new guidelines from next year.

ACC: American College of Cardiology

ADA: American Diabetic Association

ACC/ADA guidelines: published in *April 2008*
Highest risk is defined as patients with known CVD or diabetes plus one or more additional major CVD risk factor (dyslipidemia, smoking, HTN, family history)
"Highest risk" goals:
APOB < 80 mg/dl
or non-HDL cholesterol (*Tubby Factor*) < 100
or LDL-C < 70

June 14, 2008: Tim Russert has sudden death from a ruptured plaque in the coronary artery despite a normal nuclear stress test one month earlier and a LDL-C of 68 on statin. The positive calcium score and his metabolic syndrome (*Tubby syndrome*) put him at very high risk for an event. His *Tubby Factor* was elevated. This means his non-HDL cholesterol was not at the NCEP ATP III guideline goal of less than 100. This was never reported in the media to my knowledge.

American Association for Clinical Chemistry guidelines *January 2009*
Very high risk:
LDL-C < 70
non-HDL Cholesterol(*Tubby Factor*) < 80

Clinical CVD (cardiovascular disease): symptomatic disease in heart, carotids, or peripheral arteries

Subclinical vascular disease: Asymptomatic disease found by CAC (coronary artery calcium), CIMT (carotid intima-media thickness), or ankle-brachial index [taking blood pressure in leg and arm]). "Patients with documented subclinical atherosclerosis are at increased CVD risk and may be considered candidates for more aggressive therapy" (Lipoprotein Management in Patients with Cardiometabolic Risk in Diabetes Care, volume 31, number 4 [April 2008]). This is a consensus statement from the American Diabetes Association and the American College of Cardiology Foundation.

They cited the following references for this:

1. Greenland, P., et al. "Beyond Secondary Prevention: Identifying the High Risk Patient for Primary Prevention: Noninvasive Tests of Atherosclerotic Burden." *Circulation* 101 (2000):E16-E22.
2. Taylor, A. J. et al. 34th Bethesda Conference: Executive Summary—Can Atherosclerosis Imaging Techniques Improve the Detection of Patients at Risk for Ischemic Heart Disease? *Journal of the American College of Cardiology* 41 (2003):1860-1862.
3. National Cholesterol Education Program Expert Panel on Detection, Evaluation, and Treatment of High Blood Cholesterol in Adults: Executive Summary of the Third Report of the NCEP Expert Panel on Detection, Evaluation and Treatment of High Blood Cholesterol in Adults (ATP III). *JAMA* 285 (2001):2486-2497.

Lipoproteins: Particles that Transport Cholesterol and Triglycerides

1. Chylomicrons: carry triglycerides after a meal (has one APOB on it)

2. VLDL-P: carry fatty acids and triglycerides (big balls of fat that usually can't get into the wall of the artery; has one APOB on it)

3. LDL-P: carry cholesterol (has one APOB on it)

4. IDL-P (intermediate-density lipoprotein particle): has one APOB on it; can enter subendothelial space and contribute to atherosclerosis

5. Remnants-P: also come from VLDL (has one APOB on it)

Clinically Important Lipoprotein Parameters

1. **LDL-C (low-density lipoprotein cholesterol)**: major predictor of CVD. ADA/ACC guidelines state, "measurement of LDL-C may not accurately reflect the true burden of atherogenic LDL particles, especially in those with the typical lipoprotein abnormalities of CMR (cardiometabolic risk such as diabetes or metabolic [Tubby] syndrome)":

   a. Elevated triglycerides
   b. Low HDL-C
   c. Increased numbers of LDL-P

The above three findings make up *dyslipidemia*.
Often these patients have low LDL-C, which is the discordance between LDL-C and LDL-P.

2. **LDL-P (low-density lipoprotein particle)**: ADA/ACC guidelines state, "A more accurate way to capture the risk posed by LDL may be to measure the number of LDL particles directly using nuclear magnetic resonance (NMR)" (Cromwell and Otvos 2004, "Low density lipoprotein particle number and risk for cardiovascular disease," *Curr Atheroscler Rep* 6:381-387).

3. **APOB-100 (APOB)**: ADA/ACA guidelines state, "Measurements of APOB represent the total burden of particles considered most atherogenic" (Sniderman, A. D. et al. 2003, "Apolipoproteins versus lipids as indices of coronary risk and as targets for statin treatment." *Lancet* 361:777-780).

4. **Non-HDL cholesterol (Tubby Factor)**: This is the total cholesterol minus the HDL cholesterol. ADA/ACC states, "Many studies have demonstrated that non-HDL cholesterol is a better predictor of CVD risk than is LDL-C."

References given are the following:

   a. Lu, W. et al. "Non-HDL Cholesterol as a Predictor of Cardiovascular Disease in Type 2 Diabetes; the Strong Heart Study." *Diabetes Care* 26 (2003):16-23.
   b. Liu, J. et al. "Joint Distribution of Non-HDL and LDL Cholesterol and Coronary Heart Disease Risk Prediction among Individuals with and without Diabetes." *Diabetes Care* 28 (2005):1916-1921.

c.   Pischon, T. et al. "Non-High Density Lipoprotein Cholesterol and Apolipoprotein B in the Prediction of Coronary Heart Disease in Men." *Circulation* 112 (2005):3375-3383.

More from the ADA/ACC Consensus Statement, April 2008:
On page 813 from *Diabetes Care* volume 31, the following are stated:

This implies that a plasma level of 25 mg/dl LDL cholesterol would be sufficient to supply peripheral cholesterol needs.
Theoretically, all humans should maintain "newborn" LDL cholesterol levels of about 50 mg/dl to prevent atherosclerosis, and those with existing CVD should be treated to similarly low levels.

On page 817, the following are stated:

The consensus panel concludes that routine calculation and use of non-HDL cholesterol [*Tubby Factor*] constitute a better index than LDL-C for identifying high risk patients.

When both non-HDL cholesterol [*Tubby Factor*] and APOB are measured, the two are highly correlated but only moderately concordant . . . . This lack of concordance is particularly marked in patients with elevated triglyceride levels, a common finding in patients with CMR (cardiometabolic risk, including metabolic syndrome [*Tubby syndrome*]).

Because APOB appears to be a more sensitive index of residual CVD risk when LDL-C is < 130 or non-HDL cholesterol [*Tubby Factor*] is < 160 mg/dl, measurement of APOB using a standarized assay, is warranted in patients with CMR (cardiometabolic risk including metabolic syndrome [*Tubby syndrome*]) on pharmacological treatment. In particular APOB levels should be used to guide adjustments of therapy.

Triglycerides and HDL-C:
Although increased triglycerides are modestly associated with increased CVD risk, especially in women, it has been difficult to demonstrate that lowering of triglyceride level is independently

associated with a reduction in CVD events. While the HDL-C is a powerful risk predictor, the clinical trial evidence supporting treatment of low HDL-C values is modest compared with that for LDL-C lowering. For these reasons, approaches directed at lowering triglyceride-rich lipoproteins and raising reduced HDL-C level have been assigned secondary levels of therapeutic importance.

On page 818, the following is stated:

The preferred agent to use in combination with a statin is nicotinic acid (Endur-acin-Author's preference) because there is somewhat better evidence for reduction in CVD event with niacin, as monotherapy or in combination, than there is for fibrates.

Physicians need not wait for "consensus statements" to embrace new findings.

—H. Robert Superko, MD, FAHA
Circulation, May 5, 2009, p. 2404

For me, in my Topeka lipidology practice, it means the following:

1. CAC (coronary calcium score) CT scan

2. CIMT (carotid intima-media wall thickness) ultrasound

3. NMR LipoScience LipoProfile to measure LDL-P number

Lastly, never forget non-HDL-C (the poor man's APOB) is far more concordant with APOB or LDL-P than is LDL-C, but there is still a 30% discordance between non-HDL-C and LDL-P. Therefore in unusual cases like this very high risk patient, the best way to know what the actual risk is and what therapy is needed is to measure LDL-P . . . . It is too dangerous to bet one's life on lipid concentrations (LDL-C) in those with high or very high CV risk.

This is a quote from Dr. Thomas Dayspring on his blog "Lipidaholics Anonymous." It is from July 23, 2009. It is Case 239: Unusual Response to Statins.

My hope is that by the end of this book the reader will begin to understand what the above statement means. I hope my new Tubby terminology will make it a little easier to travel among the lipid jargon.

Introduction

The new health paradigm is to find subclinical atherosclerosis with coronary calcium score (CAC) and carotid intima-media thickness ultrasound so that combination therapy can be used to stabilize vulnerable plaque from inflammation and rupture and ultimately to regress the plaque that is present or at least prevent further progression of plaque.

If the coronary calcium score is one or greater and/or the carotid intima-media wall thickness shows the patient to be greater than 25% risk for a future event, we should then attempt to achieve regression of plaque as demonstrated by the repeat of the CIMT in two years.

The regression of plaque can be achieved if the following goals are achieved:

> LDL-C < 70
> Tubby Factor < 80 (also known as non-HDL cholesterol)
> LDL-P (NMR) < 750
> HDL-C > 50
> HDL-P (NMR)>35
> Triglycerides < 100
> CRPhs < 1.0
> LpPLAC normal
> APOB < 60

Getting the LDL-P < 750 or APOB < 60 is the primary and ultimate goal.
Do not lose sight of this goal.
The TG changes rapidly with diet and can be treated with more fish oil.
The HDL-C above 40 is fine if the HDL-P is above 35.
However, I doubt the new NCEP guidelines will give up on LDL-C. "It's too big to fail." To compromise, I think they will continue to use cholesterol content in the form of non-HDL cholesterol (*Tubby Factor*) even though this secondary

goal has failed to be utilized by the rank and file of physicians since the 2001 NCEP guidelines were made. I have coined the phrase Tubby Factor as that will be easier for patients and physicians to say and remember. I trade marked it in a humorous attempt to make a point. I hope my prediction fails, and APOB and LDL-P are made the primary goal.

The *cheapest* way to achieve these goals is combination therapy with generic medicine:

Simvastatin (Zocor) 10 to 40 mg at night
Endur-acin (niacin) 500 mg BID with meals
DHA/EPA fish oil 850 mg a day
Plain aspirin 325 mg, one-half tablet on Monday, Wednesday, and Friday
Vitamin D3 in oil-based capsule 1,000 to 2,000 IU a day

The *safest* way to achieve these goals is to take the following:

Crestor or Lipitor up to maximum doses
Endur-acin (niacin) 500 mg BID with meals
Lovaza (fish oil) 1,000 to 4,000 mg a day
Enteric-coated aspirin 81 mg every day (don't take with ibuprofen
    or Naprosyn)
Vitamin D3 oil-based capsules 1,000 to 2,000 IU a day

High-risk patients who want to have regression of plaque should follow the above.

I define a high-risk patient as someone in one of the following categories:

1. Subclinical atherosclerosis on CAC or CIMT
2. Known clinical atherosclerosis with myocardial infarction, plaque on duplex carotid ultrasound, aortic aneurysm
3. Diabetes mellitus
4. Metabolic syndrome
5. Two major risk factors
6. Framingham score more than or equal to 20

If you have none of the above, I still think you should have the following:

LDL-C < 100
Tubby Factor < 130
LDL particle number <1,000
Triglycerides < 150
HDL-C> 40
CRPhs < 1.0
LpPLAC normal

In a young person without risk factors but with a LDL-C more than 100, I would push diet and exercise and fish oil. Then I would consider Endur-acin 500 BID with meals.

A woman older than fifty-five years old and a man older than forty-five years old should have a CAC and a CIMT.
If either of these is positive, then they are at high risk.

A woman younger than fifty-five years old and a man younger than forty-five years old should have a CAC or CIMT if they have the following:

Father with heart disease before fifty-five years old
Mother with heart disease before sixty-five years old
BP systolic > 140
Smoking history
HDL-C < 40
TG > 200
LDL-C > 100
Tubby Factor > 130
LDL particle number > 1,000

or

Metabolic syndrome (Tubby syndrome) consists of three or more of the following:

Waist > 40 inches for men or > 35 inches for women
Sys BP > 129
Glu > 99
Triglycerides > 149
HDL-C < 50 for women or < 40 for men

I also think anyone over thirty who wants to get a baseline CAC or CIMT should do it. Young people will usually have a zero CAC. The CIMT might be more informative.

Anyone with a positive CAC or CIMT with metabolic syndrome (Tubby syndrome) is at *very high risk* for a cardiac event and should have LDL-P less than 750.
If you are not a Medicare patient or your insurance doesn't cover the NMR LipoProfile, use the standard lipid panel and calculate your Tubby Factor (non-HDL-cholesterol):

Total cholesterol
<u>minus HDL-C</u>
Tubby Factor (non-HDL cholesterol)

In a *very high-risk* patient, the goal is Tubby Factor less than 80.

Chapter One

TALE OF TWO TUBBY NEW YORKERS

Two middle-aged men with heart disease

Case One: Fat Boy from Brooklyn
4/8/91 242 lb.

Back in 1993, I had an advanced lipid testing done by the Sequoia Lipid Clinic in California. The results of this blood test were the following:

> TC (total cholesterol) 149
> LDL-C 94
> HDL-C 33
> TG (triglycerides) 157
> Small dense LDL particle size
> Lipoprotein (a) 11
> APOE 4/3.

Tubby Factor was 149 minus 33 equals 116. I did not know what non-HDL-cholesterol was back then, and it was not reported to me. It is all the cholesterol that is not HDL.

I think anybody looking at this would never have said I should be on a statin at that time. However, Dr. Robert Superko was director of the lipid institute at the time and wrote that my LDL subclass pattern B "is best treated by therapies that will lower triglycerides and increase HDL cholesterol. The first of these is appropriate diet, exercise and reduction of excess body fat. Secondary therapies include nicotinic acid and gemfibrozil. These therapies should be discussed with your physician."

At that time, nicotinic acid and gemfibrozil were very difficult to take because of flushing and constipation. I knew that from my experience with my own patients. I didn't take either medicine. I thought my total cholesterol and LDL-C were pretty good. I totally missed the point that Dr. Superko was making with me.

I did have metabolic syndrome (Tubby syndrome). Metabolic syndrome was not well known at the time. I certainly did not know about it.

10/1/95 270 lb.

9/18/1998
> Glucose 205
> Total cholesterol 154
> TG 143
> HDL-C 22
> LDL-C 103
> Tubby Factor 154-22= 132

I was found to have diabetes mellitus. I started therapeutic lifestyle changes. I didn't start diabetic medicine until I developed a neuropathy that spring.

1/09/01
> TG 227
> Total cholesterol 158
> HDL-C 29
> LDL-C 84
> Hemoglobin A1C 7.1
> Tubby factor 158-29=129

2/6/2001
I had a coronary calcium score (CAC) of 8.
I thought that was quite good.
The cardiologists in my practice said it didn't mean anything.
I was taking Lipitor.

4/21/04

>TC 127
>HDL-C 27
>LDL-C 28 (calculated; it is so low because the formula is inaccurate with TG > 200)
>TG 361
>Tubby Factor 127-27= 100 *Finally at goal*? It may have discordance with an APOB or LDL-P level. I didn't know what those were.
>Hb A1c 8.1
>Weight 260 lb.

10/19/04

Endocrinologist started me on insulin.
I weighed 269 lb.
I switched to Crestor 10 mg a day to raise my HDL-C.

12/17/04

>Hb A1c 6.8
>TC 104
>HDL-C 36
>LDL-C 77
>Tubby Factor 104-36 = 68

5/31/05

Weight 282 lb.
Waist 52 inches

1/10/2006, my calcium score (CAC) went up 125% to 20.

Clearly more needed to be done.

My 3-Hour Diet™
Success Contract

Filling out this contract will help keep you accountable to your goals. Make three copies and give them to three trusted friends who will support and motivate you in your journey to sucess.

Name: _Brian Edwards_

Today's date: _2/17/06_

I am going to weigh this many pounds: _50 lbs_

By this date: _2/17/07_

Brian Edwards
Signature

Photocopy this contract and place on your refrigerator. Join JorgeCruise.com for support and to stay accountable.

2/17/06
283 lb.

3/10/06
Weight 268 lb.
I went off insulin.

5/27/06
237 lb.

8/24/06
213 lb.
Waist 41.5 inches

7/26/2006
NMR LipoScience LipoProfile:
> LDL-P 534
> LDL-C 45
> HDL-C 54 (Notice how much my HDL-C went up with weight loss, Endur-acin, and Actos.)
> TG 124
> Total cholesterol 124
> Tubby Factor 70

6/1/2007
I also was able to get a CIMT of my carotids. Now this study is much better to follow plaque because it is just ultrasound. I won't be exposing myself to radiation any further.
The CIMT was 0.743 on my left artery. This made my artery about fifty-five years old, which is about my age. My right artery was much younger, it was in the thirty-five-year-old group, but you always use the artery that has the thicker plaque.

12/18/2007: I had lost 80 lb, and surprisingly my calcium score (CAC) went down to 1.
It is claimed in the literature that you cannot use coronary calcium score for regression purposes. It might be used to follow progression of plaque. I did change imaging machines. The prior two calcium scores were done on what is called an EBCT machine, which is probably a little more accurate than the newer machine. The third reading was done on a Siemens 64 multi-slice CT scan.

Variation in the multislice CT scan is supposed to be up to 40%. Twenty times 0.40 equals 5. That means if I had the scan the next day, the variation in score should be in the range of 15-25. My calcium score went from 20 to 1.0.

Once the calcium is in the wall, it is claimed that it does not leave. This point is not very clear to me. I was happy that my score did not continue to go up. My LDL particle number was excellent at 623. I was on Crestor.

7/28/2008 I was able to get a follow-up CIMT, and amazingly my left carotid artery thickness went from 0.74 to 0.58. This is a remarkable reduction in carotid thickness in someone who just gained 20 lb. of the 80 lb. that he lost, and who is not statin naive. The apparent improvement may be because I am APOE4, and people with this genetic makeup seem to respond extremely well to statins. These are the people who also do very badly if they continue to smoke. What's interesting is that it has been told to me that a carotid thickness of 0.3 mm is normal, and everyone's CIMT gets thicker with age, as more collagen is laid down in the wall of the artery. There are databases for manual technique CIMT. For the youngest database, which is twenty-five years old, if your CIMT is less than 0.51 mm, then you have a less than 25th percentile risk of getting an event.

Again, in full disclosure, these were different machines; I don't know if the first machine was manual or semiautomated. The second machine was semiautomated which is more accurate than manual.

7/22/08
VAP Advanced Lipid Testing Description
Direct-Measured Cholesterol Panel

Total LDL 66	LDL-R + Lp(a) + IDL
LDL-R 48	Total LDL minus Lp (a) and IDL
Lp (a) 13	more atherogenic than LDL
IDL 5	more atherogenic than LDL
Total	HDL 55 HDL2 + HDL3
HDL 2 11	Large buoyant, more protective
HDL3 44	Small dense, less protective
Total VLDL 14	VLDL1+2 and VLDL3
VLDL 1+2 4.9	Buoyant VLDL, less risk
VLDL 3 9	Dense VLDL, more risk
Total Cholesterol 135	LDL + HDL + VLDL

Secondary and Emerging Risk Factors

Triglycerides 60	linked to increased risk for CHD
Non-HDL Cholesterol 80	LDL + VLDL
Remnant lipoproteins	IDL + VLDL 3

LDL density pattern B: more risk;(A?B intermediate risk); (A: less risk)
LDL subclasses
LDL 4
LDL 3
LDL 2
LDL 1

VAP Derived apolipoproteins

APOB 100 64	*sum atherogenic lipoprotein particles most important #*
apoa1 not done	*sum anti-atherogenic lipoprotein particles*
APOB/a1 ratio not done	low ratio indicates lower risk

I think the VAP makes advanced lipid testing complicated. I prefer the NMR LipoScience LipoProfile.

Despite all the claims in the VAP descriptions, there is really one very important number: *APOB*. This is a calculated number while the immunoassay from *Berkeley HeartLab* is a directly measured APOB.

The NMR LipoScience LipoProfile also has one very important number: *LDL-P*. I think all the other information is interesting to a lipidologist, but for the patients and primary care physicians, just concentrate on getting the very high-risk patient to a goal APOB less than 60 or the LDL-P less than 750.

As Dr. Dayspring repeatedly says, once the particle number is to goal, the other numbers don't matter very much.

4/17/09
NMR LipoScience
> LDL-P 713
> LDL-C 60
> HDL-C 55
> HDL-P 37.7
> small HDL-p 26.2
> medium HDL-P 2.5
> large HDL-P 9.0
> TG 60
> TC 127
> *Tubby Factor 70*

5/6/09
VAP Advanced Lipid Testing
> *APOB 65 calculated*
> Total cholesterol 142
> TG 103
> *Tubby Factor 89*
> APOA1 154
> Total VLDL 18
> Total HDL 53
> HDL2 11
> HDL3 44
> LDL-R (real LDL) 55

9/28/09	9/28/09
NMR LipoScience	**VAP Advanced Lipid Testing**
LDL-P 761	APOB calculated 53
LDL-C 64	LDL (real) 39
HDL-C 45	HDL-C 48
HDL-P large 7.2	HDL 2 12
	HDL3 37
TG 43	TG 58
TC 118	TC 117

Tubby Factor 118-45 = 73 non-HDL cholesterol NOT 117-39 = 78? but total
LDL + VLDL = 55 + 14 = 69 (68 on report?)
VAP has made the non-HDL cholesterol more complicated.

Case Two: Big Man from Upstate New York

He was born one year before me in 1950.
In 1998, he had a calcium score of 210.
This put him at the 94% risk percentile for having an event.
He was treated to the most aggressive NCEP goal of less than 70 with Lipitor
80 g a day.

April 2008
ACC/ADA issues new guidelines for APOB.
APOB measures all the atherogenic particles. Every atherogenic particle has
one lipoprotein B on it.
The Tubby Factor (non-HDL cholesterol) tries to reflect all the cholesterol
except HDL.
The new guideline advises getting the following:
APOB < 80
Tubby Factor < 100

May 2008
LDL-C 68 (Lipitor)
TG 399 (On 2 g of niacin and TriCor 145 mg/d, compliance with niacin can be
difficult; Lovaza at 4,000 mg would have been a good addition.)
HDL-C was 37 (It had been in the 20s)
Total cholesterol 155

His Tubby Factor TM was 118. Please note that with elevated TGs, the non-HDL cholesterol has discordance with APOB.

We really don't know what is going on with his lipids here. This is why the ADA/ACC consensus advises "guiding therapy with measurements of APOB and treatment to APOB goals."

We need to know what Big Man is holding in his poker hand. It is a life-and-death bet. We need advanced lipid testing to know what cards he is holding.

Inflammation level normal with normal CRPhs.

Big Man from Upstate New York has the Tubby syndrome or the metabolic syndrome:

> Waist > 40 inches
> Glucose > 99
> BP on meds
> HDL< 40
> TG > 150

Big Man has five out of five criteria for metabolic syndrome (Tubby syndrome). The more positive criteria, the more risk and the more inflammation of the arteries. Coronary heart disease plus metabolic syndrome puts this Big Man at *very high risk* for a cardiac event.

Big Man from Upstate New York reached his primary NCEP goal of LDL-C less than 70.

He *did not reach his secondary NCEP goal* of non-HDL cholesterol (Tubby Factor) less than 100.

April 2008

The consensus statement from the American Diabetes Association and the American College of Cardiology Foundation advised the following:

> For patients with CMR (Tubby syndrome) on statin therapy, guiding therapy with measurements of APOB and treatment to APOB goals in addition to LDL-C and non-HDL cholesterol (Tubby Factor) assessments.

May 2008

Big Man was exercising and did very well on a nuclear stress test.

June 14, 2008
Big man from Buffalo dies suddenly.

Everyone was shocked when the plaque in his coronary ruptured and caused sudden death at age 58, on statins and with a negative stress test.

Why did I live and Big Man die?

I was on a path similar to him. I was on Lipitor, but when I saw that my CAC score went up 125%, I decided something more needed to be done.

A picture is worth a thousand words. Repeating the CAC clearly motivated me to lose weight and exercise and do more advanced lipid testing on myself.
I reached my LDL-C goal of less than 70, but more importantly I reached my LDL-P goal of less than 750. I did not have a NCEP ATP III secondary goal of Tubby Factor less than 100 because my TGs were not above 150. I did not let that minimum standard prevent me from treating myself more aggressively.
I believe the above paragraphs demonstrated that I had regression of plaque or at least no further progression of plaque.

I wanted to apply the principles that I used on myself to my patient population. I have accumulated data with CAC, CIMT, and NMR LipoProfile that is rather unique in the state of Kansas. This book is an analysis of that practice.

Chapter Two

FIVE WAYS TO ENHANCE A PRACTICE

Five Things to Do

1. The NMR LipoScience is a test for all the particles in the blood that are artherogenic.
2. The high-sensitivity C-reactive protein is for inflammation.
3. The CAC is a calcium score on a CT machine, either EBCT or Siemens' rapid slice.
4. The CIMT is not the traditional carotid ultrasound but the actual ultrasound of the wall thickness.
5. Use combination therapy.

1. Medicare does pay for NMR LipoScience profile. Usually three times a year is recognized practice. Most private insurance is not paying for NMR. It is $80-$100 for private pay. LDP particle number is included in this, and it is the best predictive test of events. Look at the Offspring trial data and the Framingham nested perspective trial data.

NMR LipoProfile provides data for all artherogenic particles. It also gives you the size of the LDL, which is somewhat useful. I think if the particle number is at goal, you don't have to worry too much about the size. Theoretically, the small-size LDL-P gets into the arterial wall more easily. Large-size LDL-particles are present in familial hyperlipoproteinemia which causes severe atherosclerosis. I think private-pay patients should get this test once a year to determine how much discordance their LDL-C has with LDL-P.

2. It's important to get a test for inflammation. Tim Russert died because inflammation of the artery made his plaque unstable, and this vulnerable plaque then ruptured and caused sudden death. In stroke, the ruptured plaques embolize up into the brain. Statins and fish oil lower the CRPhs. Lp-PLA2 may be a more specific test for inflammation of the arteries. I

alternate between the two tests. If the Lp-PLA2 is abnormal, I can get that three times a year as per Medicare. Otherwise, if it is normal, I only get it once a year. After I get a normal Lp-PLA2, the next time in four months, I'll get a high-sensitivity C-reactive protein. I find these studies are almost always normal as I usually have my patients on statins.

3.   CAC (calcium score) is the best test to break down patient denial. Asymptomatic patients need motivation to take medicine. Some patients are resistant to taking statins, but once I show them that they have plaque, and that any plaque can rupture and cause death, as with Tim Russert, I can usually get them to start working with me to find a statin that they can tolerate.

Secondly, I think it is important to recognize that even though everybody seems to have disease, there are some patients who have zero calcium scores even at age 90 in my practice. CAC is not used to show regression because theoretically the calcium does not leave the wall, but you certainly can use it every five years to monitor progression. However, be careful about this because of the radiation risk. If the score is 1.0 or greater, the patient has plaque. If it is greater than 400, then get a cardiology consult for further evaluation.

In my practice, I don't think I've ever had a positive nuclear stress test on someone who had a score greater than 400 without chest pain, but still I think it is something for the cardiologists to take care of. A score of zero is said to have a 99.6% likelihood of not having an event in three years. However, if you smoke, that is not true. There are many testimonials that people with zero calcium scores still have events. This is because they do have soft plaque that is not calcified yet. A patient with chest pain and a zero calcium score has a higher risk for an event.

4.   I do like the CIMT because it is an ultrasound test. It is safe, and we can repeat it frequently to monitor progression and regression of disease.

I get a CIMT if the calcium score is positive in order to monitor disease.
I get a CIMT if the calcium score is zero to see if there is disease in the carotids that is not picked up in the heart.
If there is disease in the carotid, there is probably soft plaque in the heart that is not seen by the calcium score.
I think these tests are complimentary and should both be used.

The doctor in my area, Dr. Steve Watkins, brought this modality to our region. I'd like to thank him. He put the price at $100. Insurance is not paying for this, and this is a price that just about anybody can afford.

5. Combination therapy is the way to go for safety and efficacy. High dose of statins are safe, especially with Lipitor, as in the TNT trial.

There is only a 6% decrease in LDL-C by doubling your statin.
There is a 12% decrease in LDL-C by adding 1,000 mg of niacin.
The patients get double the effect with much less risk.

Simvastatin 80 mg is high risk in terms of developing rhabdomyolysis. If disease is present or if there is plaque in the coronaries with the calcium score positive or atheromas in the carotids with a thick CIMT, I like to be very aggressive and get the particle number less than 750 in order to achieve regression. Generic simvastatin is $10 for three months' supply.

Endur-acin at 500 mg BID with meals will rarely cause flushing. It costs $70 for 1,000 tabs on the Internet. Simply google Endur-acin to find the site.

Chapter Three

THE TREATMENT OF A PATIENT AS MY KNOWLEDGE OF LIPID IMPROVES

My Experience from My Practice

5/28/03

Sixty-five-year-old male diagnosed with hyperlipidemia by his previous primary care physician

Significant weight loss since surgery and had been able to stop BP meds

TG 315

Total cholesterol 177

HDL-C 30

LDL-C 84

Instructions: continue low-fat, low-cholesterol diet

Follow-up: yearly and sooner prn

ATP III states the following:

Treatment of TG >150:

Lose weight

Exercise

If triglycerides was more than 200 after LDL goal was reached, set secondary goal for non-HDL cholesterol (Tubby Factor) 30 mg/dl higher that LDL goal.

(100 + 30 = 130) Patients with CHD or CHD equivalent (FRS > 20%)

(130 + 30 = 160) Patients with 2+ risk factors and 10 year risk FRS < 21%

Total cholesterol 177

subtract HDL—30

non-HDL cholesterol (Tubby Factor) 147

"If triglycerides 200-499 mg/dl after LDL goal is reached, consider adding drug if needed to reach non-HDL cholesterol goal (Tubby Factor) by intensifying therapy with LDL-lowering drug or add niacin or fibrate to further lower VLDL."

This primary care physician did not have to medically treat this high TG with drugs as per the guidelines. That is, if I understand the above guidelines.

12/10/04
I saw this sixty-five-year-old male for the first time.
Weight 174 lb., waist 92 cm.
Risk factors for CAD include age > 45 years old
I told him to take a baby aspirin every day.

> Lab 12/10/04
> TC 156
> LDL-C 89
> TG 215
> HDL-C 24
> Glu 95

4/06
"Patient had lipid panel on 12/10/04. At that time LDL-C was low at 89 but he also had a poor HDL-C to triglyceride ratio suggesting metabolic syndrome (Tubby Syndrome)."
Started on one fish oil tab

Step 8 of the ATP III guidelines states to identify metabolic syndrome and treat if present after three months of therapeutic lifestyle changes.
Treat elevated triglycerides and/or low HDL as above.

8/06
Patient was tolerating omega-3 fish oil 1,000 mg a day. It had raised his LDL-C (93) a little bit.

Added Endur-acin 500 mg QHS.
Check glucose, AST, TG, and HDL in two months.

10/19/2006
I attended my first lipid management training course in Kansas City.

Up to this point, I did not know the fine points of the NCEP ATP III guidelines. I did not even know what the non-HDL cholesterol was.
I did not realize that one tab of fish oil and one tab of niacin would do very little for triglycerides.

1/23/07
"Patient comes in today to follow up on his metabolic syndrome."
AST 31, glucose 99, HDL-C 28, LDL-C 83, TG 268
Increased Endur-acin to 500 mg twice a day, increased fish oil to two tabs a day

Calculated *Framingham risk score* (FRS) so I could order a CAC

AGE 67	11 points
Total Cholesterol 148	0 points
HDL < 40	2 points
BP sys 160 untreated	2 points (he says his BP is 110 at home)
No smoking	0 points
Total	15 points Framingham risk is 20%
	(Intermediate risk)

In Kansas, Medicare will pay for a CAC CT for patients with FRS 10-20% if he has an equivocal stress test (non-nuclear).

5/24/07

> TG 346
> HDL-C 30
> AST 45 (was 31)

Patient said he was taking Niaspan 500 mg a day.
I did not increase niacin because glucose went up to 106 (it was 99). He now has prediabetes.
He still was only taking one fish oil a day, and I now increased it to three fish oil a day.
Patient's stress treadmill was equivocal so we will send him for a CAC.

At this time, I was very concerned about increasing the insulin resistance in metabolic syndrome patients. I had found small changes in the fasting glucose mean very little, and indeed the Hb A1c did not change on 1 g of niacin. Now

I go right to Endur-acin 500 mg BID with meals as there is almost no flushing, and the glucose has not been an issue.

6/04/07
CAC 186

"Based on this the patient clearly has coronary artery disease. Since the patient is now in high risk as per Framingham score, will do the optimal recommendation of getting LDL-C under 70."

10/25/07
DX:
1. Coronary artery disease (CAC 186)
2. Metabolic syndrome
3. Prediabetes
4. Hyperlipidemia
5. Framingham risk score 20%

Switch fish oil to Lovaza TID

3/27/08
Crestor 5 mg a day

I don't know why it took me ten months to get statin started. Often the patient is resistant to starting statins.

7/29/08
Patient told me he is on *no-flush niacin*. I told him this is inactive on lipids.
I started Endur-acin 500 mg BID.
Crestor decreased to 5 mg QOD as LDL-C was 58.

12/2/08
Crestor 5 mg every other day
Endur-acin 500 mg BID
Fish oil three tabs a day
Aspirin 81 mg a day
Vitamin D 1,000 IU a day

4/03/09
Advised CIMT for $100 so we can follow patient for progression or regression of atheroma of the carotids

7/31/09

CIMT was *0.54 mm* which is less than 25th percentile of other men his age.

The other "low" HDL-C patient was a seventy-year-old man with LDL-P of 622 on Crestor 5 mg and Endur-acin 500 mg BID. His HDL-C was 33, and his HDL-P was 26.1 with 21.6 small HDL-P. Again a surprise on the small number of large HDL-P in a patient on niacin. His TG was 105. I thought I would again follow Dr. Dayspring's advice. If his LDL-P was at goal, the HDL-C and the TG level did not matter. He quoted the NCEP guidelines, "In patients with high TG (between 200 and 500 mg/dl) the NCEP goal of therapy is LDL-C and non-HDL-C (the Tubby Factor); NCEP would state *case closed* despite the still low HDL-C and high TG." The patient in this case had a Tubby Factor of 59 and an LDL-C of 16, so NCEP would say case closed despite the TG of 217 and the HDL-C of 24.

Step 2 of ATP III guidelines states to identify presence of *clinical* atherosclerotic disease that confers high risk for coronary artery disease events (CHD risk equivalent).

This is the paradigm shift that is needed. The guidelines should state to identify *subclinical* atherosclerosis in patients with one risk factor or the metabolic syndrome (Tubby syndrome).

I look at this history and realize that the Tubby plan would have saved a lot of time and made a diagnosis immediately. If the patient had a CAC back in 2003, he would have been on a statin much sooner. I had not started a statin because the LDL-C was below 100. If I had done an NMR LipoProfile, I would have seen that his LDL-P was elevated. Medicare was not paying for NMR LipoScience LipoProfiles or CAC's back in December 2004. CAC and CIMT find subclinical atherosclerosis. The Tubby guidelines advise getting the Tubby Factor (non-HDL cholesterol) less than 80 in very high-risk patients. This turned out to be a very high-risk patient as he had coronary artery disease and the metabolic syndrome (Tubby syndrome). He was not started on a statin from May 28, 2003 until March 27, 2008. That is almost five years without statins. Statins not only lower LDL-C and LDL-P, they also decrease inflammation. This patient had five years risk of rupturing his coronary plaque without treatment. Why do the guidelines tolerate that? Why are the guidelines so complicated that a TG of more than 300 is only treated with diet and exercise which patients usually don't comply with. I couldn't even get this patient to increase his fish oil for months or take the active niacin. If he knew in 2003 that he had a plaque that might cause sudden death, he would have been more compliant with the medications. There is so much confusion with the guidelines that definitive action is not taken. The language is beyond people and physicians. To tell a patient they have metabolic syndrome and thus their non-HDL cholesterol is probably elevated while their LDL-C is normal is too much verbiage. This is why I have coined the term Tubby Factor. A patient can walk into the office and ask for his Tubby Factor (non-HDL cholesterol) because he thinks he has the Tubby syndrome. He just has to look in the mirror to suspect he has the Tubby syndrome. At this point, a CAC and a CIMT can be ordered to determine risk assessment. The Framingham risk score is burdensome and underestimates the risk. It is easy for a patient to understand that a plaque can rupture and cause death as the first symptom. The Tubby guidelines are easy to do and for everyone to understand.

The ATP III guidelines already allow ordering a CAC or CIMT or CRPhs on a patient with FRS of 10-20 %. It is okay to order CAC/CIMT for women with less than 10% risk. I don't think I am too radical to change this guideline to go right to the imaging so we can know immediately what cards the patient is holding in this game of life or death poker.

In the text *Management of Lipids in Clinical Practice* (sixth edition) by Neil Stone and Conrad Blum, on page 373, there is a clinical tip:

> Risk assessment using the Framingham risk score for "hard" CHD becomes less reliable in older patients, especially men, as age alone plays such a strong role in determining global risk. Clinicians may find measurement of sub-clinical atherosclerosis useful in the decision to treat more intensively. For example, and EBCT (CAC) calcium score in the upper 25th percentile for age, an abnormal CIMT, or an abnormal ankle-brachial index may suggest lower goals (hence intensive lipid-lowering therapy) may be appropriate (ATP III report 2001).

In the text *Clinical Challenges in Lipid Disorders* by Peter Toth and Domenic Sica, on page 57, I learned about the SHAPE trial:

> The Screening for Heart Attack Prevention and Education (SHAPE) task force recently recommended screening for subclinicial

atherosclerosis using computed tomography (CAC), carotid artery ultrasound, or both, for all asymptomatic "at risk" men aged 45-75 years and women aged 55-75 years old. The SHAPE trial considered a positive test for atherosclerosis a CAC > or equal to one, or CIMT > or equal to 50th percentile or presence of carotid plaque. However, those considered high risk or CHD equivalent were further subcategorized as having a CAC > 100 or >75th percentile or a CIMT > or equal to 1.0 mm or > 75th percentile. These individuals would be treated to the same goals as high risk CHD equivalent patients from the NCEP-ATP III guidelines.

Finally, in my education, I read from the National Lipid Association Self-Assessment Program critique book (volume one) on page 108:

NCEP ATP III does not recommend measurement of emerging risk factors during an initial evaluation. However, NCEP ATP III provides examples of where measurement of these factors may be useful including:

1- to elevate a patient with multiple CHD risk factors and an estimated 10 yr risk of < 20% to a CHD risk equivalent status
2- to guide use of LDL-C lowering drugs in patients with < 2 risk factors and a LDL-C between 160 and 189 mg/dl.
3- to improve the assessment in middle-aged and older patients in whom traditional risk factors may have declined in predictive power.

(Expert Panel on Detection, Evaluation, and Treatment of High Blood Cholesterol in Adults, Executive summary of the third report of the National Cholesterol Education Program [NCEP] Expert Panel on Detection, Evaluation, and Treatment of High Blood Cholesterol in Adults [Adult Treatment Panel III], *JAMA* 2001, f285:2486-2497)

Around January 2007, Kansas Medicare began paying for CACs in patients with FRS 10-20% with an equivocal stress test.
Since then I have had about 150 CACs done that were paid for by Medicare.
Then Medicare began paying for NMR LipoScience LipoProfiles. I began doing those routinely.

The result are the spreadsheets in of the book.

I have also had more than one hundred patients pay $200 on their own for CAC as their private insurance will not pay for it.

Most private insurance companies will not pay for NMR LipoScience LipoProfile. For these patients, I advise calculating the Tubby Factor from the standard lipid profile.

Chapter Four

THE POKER HAND

Diagnosing atherosclerosis in a patient is like playing poker.

We ask the patient about his major risk factors.

Many patients are very health conscious and don't smoke.

The family history is often thought to be positive, but if the father did not have an event before fifty-five years old or the mother before sixty-five years old, it is negative. Siblings count as well.

If the patient is male and more than forty-four years old or female and more than fifty-four years old, the patient has a positive risk factor.

So far, this was a forty-five-year-old male patient with no smoking history and whose father had a heart attack at fifty-four years old.

One risk factor positive so far. We knew one of the five cards in the patient's poker hand.

We were in the doctor's office, so it was "easy" to find out the next card. Was the systolic blood pressure 140 or greater? It was 139. The patient said whenever he takes it outside of the doctor's office, it is less than 130 systolic. We were back to guessing at the cards.

We got a blood test on this Tubby patient, and it showed an HDL-C of 41, negative for risk factor. HDL-C is the least reliable of the lipid tests. The repeat HDL-Cs might range from 37 (positive risk factor) to 45 (negative risk factor). It was like the blood pressure, we were guessing at what the patient was holding in his poker hand. He said he would diet and exercise. Now we knew he was bluffing.

The Framingham risk score is what primary care physicians are told to figure out on their patients. This patient only had one risk factor, and NCEP ATP III guidelines state we don't need to get it. We want to know what the patient's poker hand was, so we figured it out anyway. After all, the poker bet is life and death.

FRS

Age 45 years old	3 points
Total cholesterol 162	2 points
Nonsmoker	0 points
HDL 41	1 point
Systolic BP 139	1 point
Total points	7 points

Framingham risk score is 3% risk over the next ten years.

This had not helped much. If anything, we thought the patient was holding a good poker hand and going to live the next ten years.

However, this book is about the Tubby Factor. We saw this patient had apple-shaped obesity, so we checked him for the Tubby syndrome (metabolic syndrome).

Waist 41 inches	(+)
BP systolic 139	(+)
HDL 41	(-)
TG 149	(-)
Fasting glucose 99	(-)

No Tubby syndrome. Only two of the five criteria are positive.

The Tubby Factor is 162 minus 41 equals 121.

Since this patient appeared to be low risk, the Tubby Factor or non-HDL cholesterol was considered normal by NCEP standards. Since the TGs are less than 200, they would not even ask us to calculate the Tubby Factor.

I guess we were done. It looked like the patient had a winning poker hand. Of course, we would tell him to lose weight and follow therapeutic lifestyle changes.

Wait a second. This is 2009. Tim Russert had a CAC CT in 1998. We have a way to know exactly what the patient's poker hand is. This is a life and death wager after all.

In my town, it costs $200. Medicare covers some patients. Private insurance doesn't cover anyone.

His CAC calcium score is 99. This proves the patient has plaque, but some would say it does not elevate him to the next risk category. They claim it has to be over 100. I myself believe the patient is now high risk and needs to get his LDL-P less than 1,000 or less than 750 if we want to show regression.

Just to know exactly all the cards the patient is holding, I ordered a CIMT and NMR LipoScience LipoProfile. Each cost $100.

The CIMT showed a carotid wall thickness of 1.00 mm and puts him in the 75th percentile range. *Wow!*

The NMR shows an LDL-P of 1,400. I want to get his LDL-P less than 750 and show regression in two years with repeat CIMT.

This is how we play poker in Topeka. No more guessing about the player's hand. Find the subclinical (no symptoms) atherosclerosis and stabilize it and prevent rupture and sudden death.

Chapter Five

HIDDEN RISK

pt #	Age	sex	DM	Met Syn	CAC	CIMT	cimt%	Carotid Stenosis	LDLp	NON-HDL	LDLc	HDL	TG	Total CHOL	Statin	Enduracin	Zetia	Wel/Tri
	58	F		5	70				4071	281	221	48	301	329				
3	76	F			+CATH			59	3656	331	N/C	53	435	384				WEL
3	75	F							3125	269	196	55	363	324				
	75	F							3039	314	237	38	384	352				
	70	F							2705	207	129	42	391	249				
	52	F	Y						2698	229	202	61	137	290	C20			W
	92	F			391			39	2670	264	217	54	236	318	C10			
31	61								2580	221	178	68	215	289				
	68								2473	185	136	84	245	269				
13	56	F	Y	5					2452	194	162	40	158	234				
	62								2431	198	166	37	161	235				
	65	F	Y						2428	328	N/C	46	1243	374				
	69	F	Y	4					2415	188	161	45	133	233				
	67	F		3		0.7	50	NORMAL	2398	230	185	61	226	291				
	79	M			+CATH			39	2322	216	158	36	291	252	C5/O	Y		
37	38								2296	219	181	12	188	231				
	66								2271	211	169	38	210	249				
	59								2259	209	189	44	102	253				
	66	M			1				2254	187	137	33	252	220	PRA40			
	53	F				0.67	50		2249	171	147	55	156	226				
30	89								2246	198	173	53	126	251				
3	75	F							2245	233	181	68	258	301				
	61	M		5					2242	205	138	36	333	241				
	61	M	Y						2213	206	181	35	124	241		Y		W
31	61								2196	168	134	43	172	211				
	60								2188	256	N/C	69	599	325				
13	57	F	Y	5					2157	150	129	41	103	191				
	72	F							2151	183	156	53	140	236	C10			
	58	M	Y					10	2146	158	98	43	302	201	C5			TRI
	77	F			0	1.04	>75		2141	160	140	50	100	210		Y		W/TRI
	62	M							2135	195	120	61	376	256				
	52	F	Y		0				2118	215	169	53	229	268				
	77	M		3					2108	171	141	33	148	204				
	47								2087	215	174	57	203	272				
17	75	M							2086	201	152	40	243	241				
	47								2075	199	161	40	190	239				
17	76	M						40	2072	172	129	39	213	211	LES80	Y		
30	89								2071	258	226	51	160	309				
37	39								2063	159	N/C	41	437	200				
	49								2044	194	N/C	42	448	236				
	54	M	Y						2021	121	99	32	110	153				
	79								2020	148	129	54	96	202				
	66	F							2020	209	189	54	100	263				
	75	F	Y	5	+CATH				2017	254	204	53	249	307	L10/O	Y		
	48	M		3	0	0.63	50		2007	133	111	40	108	173				
	75								2007	222	189	44	165	266				
	88	F							2007	128	115	57	64	185				

Age	sex	DM	Met Syn	CAC	CIMT	cimt%	Carotid Stenosis	LDLp	NON-HDL	LDLc	HDL	TG	Total CHOL	Statin	Enduracin	Zetia	Wel/Tri
77	M	Y		+CATH			39	722	80	8	43	360	123	L40	Y	Y	TRI
3 DRUG																	
66	M			+CATH	0.832		39	492	45	37	67	41	112	C40	Y	Y	
63	M	Y		+CATH			9	555	124	45	40	395	164	S20	Y	Y	
76	M			+CATH			39	694	63	45	63	91	126	C40	Y	Y	
90	M	Y		+CATH			80	697	66	19	37	234	103	S20	Y	Y	
76	M	Y		+CATH			39	700	45	32	44	64	89	L80	Y	Y	
78	M			460			9	714	57	51	67	30	124	S20	Y	Y	
79	M	Y		1500			39	738	39	31	48	41	87	C40	Y	Y	
74	M	Y		+CATH			59	749	47	35	80	61	127	S40	Y	Y	
2 DRUG																	
57	M			0	0.99	>75		439	77	39	61	191	138	C10	Y		
71	F			523			59	487	68	60	97	42	165	C10	Y		
75	M		5	127			49	559	60	40	53	100	113	C20	Y		
67	M		4	2	0.67	<25		605	73	55	68	88	141	C20	Y		
68	F	Y		2751			59	655	81	61	65	99	146	C20	Y		
83	M			1700			39	659	84	74	86	52	170	C10	Y		
72	M	Y		+CATH			9	665	66	23	58	214	124	C20	Y		
68	F			+CATH			39	697	80	59	68	148	148	C10	Y		
78	M	Y					39	718	63	46	43	87	106	C10	Y		
82	F	Y					49	737	76	56	81	101	157	C10	Y		
69	M			POS	0.79	50		598	66	53	54	64	120	C5	N1000		
70	M			186	0.54	<25		622	64	43	33	105	97	C5	Y		
92	F			374			9	623	66	52	58	71	124	C5/O	Y		
73	M			20	0.72	50	39	678	68	57	57	56	125	C5	Y		
84	F		4	33	0.83	50		509	81	65	91	78	172	L20	Y		
71	M			+CATH			9	581	97	59	53	192	150	L10	Y		
83	F			+CATH			49	637	60	47	57	64	117	L80	Y		
95	M			104			39	660	56	50	43	31	99	L10	Y		
57	M	Y		+CATH				672	63	52	43	53	106	L20	NIA		
54	M			0	0.58	<25		676	66	46	44	100	110	L10	Y		
72	M			1042				679	66	51	50	76	116	L10	Y		
89	F			+			39	749	78	63	74	75	152	L40	Y		
71	F		2	0	0.62	<25		732	82	70	76	61	158	P40	Y		
81	F						59	736	82	69	83	65	165	PRA40	Y		
73	M	Y					9	363	50	42	69	42	119	S40	Y		
87	M						39	456	52	44	57	40	109	S40	Y		
79	M			+ CATH			9	588	50	43	48	37	98	S40	Y		
88	M			+			39	591	53	36	40	87	93	S20	Y		
75	F						39	645	71	51	63	98	134	S40	Y		
77	M						9	649	59	51	58	39	117	S40	Y		
88	F			+			39	694	92	21	44	354	136	S40	Y		
62	M	Y		+CATH			39	695	70	53	42	85	112	S20	Y		
64	M			4				714	81	62	65	95	146	S40	Y		
69	M			12			NORMAL	714	84	68	74	82	158	S40	Y		
80	F						9	745	75	64	86	54	161	C10		Y	
85	M			AAA			9	705	55	41	86	68	141	C20		Y	
64	M	Y		+CATH	1.05	>75	9	716	85	59	68	130	153	C20		Y	
57	F	Y	5					730	44	28	51	82	95	C5		Y	
68	M			+ CATH			39	294	53	44	89	47	142	L10		Y	
55	F	Y		+CATH				517	48	33	65	75	113	S10		Y	
86	M			+CATH			39	734	61	54	53	34	114	S20		Y	
79	F			309				653	64	54	73	52	137	S40		Y	
51	F							620	67	58	72	45	139	S40		Y	
71	F			+			positive	728	71	48	58	115	129	S80		Y	
50	F	Y	5		0.55	50		681	107	71	53	180	160	S40			W
1 DRUG																	
86	F			+CATH				586	71	54	72	83	143	C10			
85	F	Y		0.9			39	594	83	72	74	54	157	C10			
88	F			841			49	690	69	52	58	83	127	C20			
68				+cath				745	77	60	85	84	162	C10			
48	F	Y			0.54	50		381	60	39	71	107	131	C5			
52	M			3871	0.57	<25		401	68	46	98	111	166	C5			
80	F	Y		+CATH			9	462	52	27	61	126	113	C5			
59	F			73	0.87	>75		639	83	71	74	59	157	C5			
72	F			11			9	640	84	60	75	118	159	C5			
79	F			232			39	661	95	74	66	107	161	C5			
55								674	64	54	68	51	132	C5			

My database is the only one of its kind in Kansas. To my knowledge, I am the only physician to combine CAC, CIMT, and NMR LipoScience LipoProfile on many of my patients.

The practice has been amazing in the number of patients who thought they were healthy, only to find they have vulnerable plaque.

This is evident in three areas of testing.

1. CIMT had more than 75th percentile in eleven patients with a CAC of zero.
2. CAC had thirteen number of positive results in patients with CIMT of less than 25th percentile risk
3   Twenty-two patients had LDL-C of less than 160 or unable to calculate when in fact their LDL-P was more than 2,000.

I started my education in lipidology on October 19, 2006, at the Intercontinental Hotel in Kansas City, Missouri, by taking a lipid management training course sponsored by the National Lipid Association.

I passed my lipidology boards in Chicago in September 2008.

I was elected to the Midwest Lipid Association board at the NLA meeting in Cincinnati 2009.

I have enclosed data demonstrating my work over the last two years with CAC (coronary artery calcium), CIMT (carotid intima-media thickness) and the advance lipid testing by NMR LipoScience LipoProfile.

The most amazing fact is that I uncovered hidden disease and risk, which would have been missed with the routine lipid panel.

The CIMT showed eleven patients that had more than 75th percentile risk with a calcium score of zero.

The CAC had a positive calcium score in thirteen patients with CIMT at less than 25th percentile risk.

The LDL-P was more than 2,000 in twenty-two patients with LDL-C less than 160.

Forty-six patients that we can prevent further progression of disease with combination therapy.

This spreadsheet includes data from the following sources:

1. **CAC**—calcium scores of patients. A score of one or greater means they have coronary plaque
2. **CIMT**—done by Dr. Watkins. It is interpreted at three risk levels:

   More than 75th percentile risk
   More than 25th to 75th percentile risk which I abbreviate at 50th percentile risk
   Less than 25th percentile risk

3. NMR LipoScience LipoProfile. This gives the LDL particle number (LDL-P). This is the test most predictive of cardiovascular disease. In my opinion, it has replaced LDL-C and Non-HDL cholesterol. Therapy given with **S** = simvastatin, **C** = Crestor, **L** = Lipitor, **Pra** = pravastatin

Chapter Six

THE METABOLIC SYNDROME (TUBBY SYNDROME)

This can also be called the Tubby syndrome. This is what causes the increased Tubby Factor in America. The Tubby syndrome is much more useful than the Framingham risk score, which does not include waist or triglycerides or glucose level, in determining risk.

If one of my patients has plaque as demonstrated by CAC or CIMT and also has metabolic syndrome, I tell him he has a very high risk of a cardiac event in his lifetime. It can be prevented if we get the LDL-P less than 750 by giving simvastatin/Endur-acin.

The above is the Tubby plan. It is so simple.

This is the new paradigm of preventive medicine in America. Find subclinical atherosclerosis at an early age and then prevent it from progressing. I do CIMTs every two years to make certain we are not missing something in the patient's total picture. If there is progression of atheroma in the carotid, then a closer look at the patient is needed.

Simvastatin and Endur-acin are less than $90 a year.

Once the above is done, I think the patient becomes more engaged and will then start the life-long TLC or the Tubby lifestyle changes.

NCEP advised TLC (therapeutic lifestyle change) first. That gives the patient a year to indulge in denial. The physician also is deluded in thinking he has offered the patient a real change.

NCEP had it backward in terms of clinical practice. A patient must know that he has vulnerable plaque, which is subject to inflammation and may rupture to cause sudden death, as a first sign of disease.

We have many poster boys for sudden death, Tim Russert, the comedian Bernie Mac, Jim Fixx the runner, etc.

Once a patient sees progress in his numbers, then the visualization of success is more real. He can change. Now he must exercise and lose some weight. This will treat his metabolic syndrome. This will treat the inflammation. It will lower his CRPhs to 0.02.

The fat in the belly (Tubby fat) secretes many chemicals that inflame the arteries. This makes the membrane covering the plaque in the artery unstable. Inflamed and unstable, the membrane is likely to rupture and cause sudden death.

Hs-CRP and Lp-PLA2 are two blood tests to check for inflammation. The JUPITER trial was supposedly done on healthy people. This is why the FDA allowed Crestor to be given against placebo. Many of the patients had metabolic syndrome (Tubby syndrome). They had "normal" LDL-C of less than 130.

It turns out because so many patients had the Tubby syndrome, there was discordance with the APOB (LDL-P) in the JUPITER trial. The average APOB was at a high-risk level. The JUPITER trial was done on people with high CRPhs. They had elevated CRPhs because most of them had the Tubby syndrome.

Five Criteria for Tubby Syndrome:

> 1—Apple obesity (waist > 40 inches for men and > 35 inches for women)
> 2—Pre-diabetes (fasting glucose > 99)
> 3—Fasting Triglycerides > 149
> 4—Systolic Blood Pressure > 129 or already on hypertension medicine.
> 5—HDL< 40 for men and < 50 for women

If a patient has three or more of the above, they are diagnosed with Metabolic (Tubby syndrome).

Chapter Seven

GUIDELINES ARE TOO COMPLICATED

Newsflash: Even the *NEJM* could not calculate the Framingham risk score correctly in its September 9, 2009, case study. They have proven my point that simply getting a CAC/CIMT will tell a patient and a doctor that the patient is at high risk and should be treated aggressively.

The guidelines put forth by NCEP/ATP III are just way too complicated.

The Tubby guideline is so simple: Get the Tubby Factor (non-HDL cholesterol) less than 80.

Use the Tubby plan to get there:

1. Get a CAC (calcium score)   (a CT scan costs $100 to $400)
2. Get a CIMT   (a ultrasound test $100 to $200)
3. Get a NMR-P blood level   (a blood test from LipoScience $100)
4. Combination therapy   (simvastatin/Endur-acin for less than $90 a year)

Or you can try to figure out the present guidelines.
A short list of guidelines:

1. Major risk factors
2. Framingham risk score (FRS)
3. NECP/ATP
4. Metabolic syndrome
5. Cardiovascular equivalents
6. Emerging risk factors
7. American Diabetic Association guidelines
8. American Heart Association guidelines
9. ACC/ADA consensus report guidelines April 2008

Now I'd like the doctors to name the five major risk factors.

Very few can nail the family history category. I have a cue card on my computer to remind me. A doctor will say that he does this in his head, but that really isn't sufficient when we talk about electronic medical records and trying to document risk for the federal government.

Allow me to summarize the ATP III guidelines on the At-A-Glance Quick Desk Reference:

1. Determine lipoprotein levels. (It turns out they mean cholesterol content, so it is already confusing.)
    LDL-C of less than 100 is optimal. This means it is associated with a very low risk of atherosclerosis.
2. Identify presence of clinical atherosclerotic disease. This means, do they have symptoms of disease or signs of aneurysm (AAA)?
3. Major risk factors present
    (curious add-on: subtract one risk factor if HDL-C is greater than 60)
4. If two major risk factors or more are present, determine Framingham risk score (FRS).
5. Determine Risk Category for ten-year period   Begin drug therapy:

High risk is FRS > 20% or cardiac equivalent	If LDL-C > 129
Intermediate risk is FRS 20% to > 9%	If LDL-C > 129
Low risk is FRS 9% or less	If LDL-C > 159
Only one major risk factor or less	If LDL-C >189

6. Initiate therapeutic lifestyle changes (TLC) for LDL-C

High risk	> 99
Intermediate risk	> 129
Low risk	> 129
One or less risk factor	> 159

The problem with this is that the Tubby syndrome is well known to often have LDL-C of less than 100. Later they try to address this.

7   Consider adding drug therapy with TLC as per LDL-C levels in step 5 if cardiac equivalent.

For intermediate risk and lower, do TLC for three months first.

8. If metabolic syndrome (Tubby syndrome) is still present after three months of TLC, treat it.

    [1]- Treat blood pressure
    [2]- Give aspirin for cardiac heart disease
    [3]- Treat elevated TG as in next step
    [4]- Treat low HDL-C as in next step

9. Treat elevated triglycerides.
    Treat everyone with TG > 499

Secondary goal of NCEP:
"If triglycerides are > 199 after LDL-C goal is reached, set secondary goal for *non-HDL* cholesterol (total minus HDL) 30 mg/dl higher than LDL-C goal."
It is difficult to believe that not treating a TG of 498 is acceptable if the Tubby Factor is less than 100.

I probably made some errors in my interpretation. I have only been studying these rules intensely since my first course in Kansas City in October 2006. I did pass my lipidology boards in September 2008. This only goes to show that the average primary care provider may have a difficult time with understanding these guidelines. The *NEJM* got the FRS wrong in September 2009. We need something simple.

Framingham Risk Score (FRS)

The FRS is the bedrock of evidence-based medicine for the NCEP/ATP guidelines.

It consists of the following:

> age
> total cholesterol
> smoking
> HDL
> blood pressure

I am proposing to simplify risk stratification by ordering CAC/CIMT. It's simple. If you have plaque, you are high risk.

If you have Tubby syndrome and plaque, you are very high risk, and you want your LDL-P less than 750.

Very few physicians take the time to score the patients with the above five categories.
The FRS is very flawed in today's Tubby society. It leaves out waist size, TG, and glucose.
It also leaves out family history and was done on a white northeastern USA population.
The HDL-C< 40, makes some sense, but to subtract a point if HDL-C is greater than 60 may not make much sense unless they switch it to HDL-P.
Blood pressure readings are so variable. Have the patient take them at home first thing in the morning and average it out?
The FRS is to be calculated on lab results before taking statins. Nowadays, that is not always easy.

I have been doing the Framingham risk score for my patients because Kansas Medicare will pay for their CAC if they are intermediate risk and have an equivocal treadmill stress test or are unable to do the treadmill.

Intermediate risk means the chance of having a heart attack or stroke in ten years is from 10 to 20%. This means 1-2% per year. That means one in one hundred people to one in fifty people will have an event. This is not lifetime risk.

I think some people hear their risk is one in one hundred and figure they like those odds enough that they will not take statins.

My practice of medicine is on individuals. If I get a CAC/CIMT and they are positive, the patient is elevated to high risk.

I say make the guidelines based on what is best for the individual patient and is easy to understand. This is what I have done in my practice.

Since 2001, the NCEP secondary guideline is to get the non-HDL cholesterol to goal if TG is more than 200 after treating the LDL-C to goal.

Make it simple. Get everybody with plaque on CAC/CIMT to Tubby Factor less than 80.

In 2001, the NCEP/ATP guidelines said to get LDL-C less than 100 in high-risk patients.

After Prove-it trial, the physicians were given the option to get their patients to LDL-C of less than 70. They could not make it a hard-and-fast rule because that would have disrupted several trials that were going on at the time.
Anyway, in 2004, they did their best, and they said if you are very high risk, (which means you have CHD plus some other things that I'll get into later) then it's the option of the doctor to try to get the LDL-C under 70. Now let's emphasize this point, "the option of the physician." Clearly a physician uses these guidelines as the *minimum* to treat patients. If he has any concern, he should go on and treat them aggressively.

These are the coronary heart disease equivalents or high-risk equivalents:

1. Symptomatic carotid disease
2. Clinical coronary heart disease
3. Peripheral artery disease
4. Abdominal aortic aneurysm
5. Diabetes mellitus (plus one major risk factor?)
6. FRS > 20%
7. CAC > 99
8. CIMT > 50% risk
9. CRPhs 2.0

To be very high risk, a patient must have one of the six above and one of the four below:

1. Metabolic syndrome (Tubby syndrome)
2. Acute coronary syndrome
3. Several poorly controlled risk factors
4. Multiple risk factors (especially diabetes mellitus)

In my zeal to prevent sudden death in my patients, I have decided to use CAC 1.0 or greater and CIMT more than 25% to be cardiac equivalent.
I will treat these patients to LDL-P of less than 1,000 or a Tubby Factor of less than 100 if they don't want aggressive therapy.
My preference is to get them to LDL-P of less than 750 or Tubby Factor less than 80 to get regression of the atheroma on the CIMT in two years.

If they also have Tubby syndrome and thus are *very high risk*, I will aggressively get their LDL-P less than 750 or their Tubby Factor less than 80 or their APOB less than 60.

Circ 2004;110:231

I would recommend looking at the ADA-ACC recent guidelines in March 2008, which recommend using APOB levels or LDL particle numbers instead of simply using LDL-C levels. As my professors have said, guidelines are similar to the story in *Ghostbusters*. Bill Murray saw Sigourney Weaver as a client. She was possessed. She tried to get him in bed. He told her, "It's usually a hard fast rule of mine not to go to bed with people possessed." She takes off her dress, he looks, he says, "It's more of a guideline." With that, let me go on to say that the new guidelines from NCEP-ATP III are coming out very soon. I think that as it is often said that as soon as a guideline is made, it is often out of date. Another professor of mine said that he did a study, and the profession that has the longest longevity are physicians. They have access to health care, they take the medicine, they have access to it. They have access to taking their blood pressure. They live longer than anyone else. This is in contrast to the old days, when they used to go around and meet everyone with infections before antibiotics.

Chapter Eight

GOALS

Population Distributions of LDL-C, non-HDL-C, ApoB and LDL-P in Framingham Offspring Study

Percentile	LDL-C (mg/dL)	Non-HDL-C (mg/dL)	LDL-P (nmol/L)	ApoB (mg/dL)
2	70	83	720	54
5	78	94	850	62
10	88	104	940	69
20	100	119	1100	78
30	111	132	1220	85
40	120	143	1330	91
50	130	153	1440	97
60	139	163	1540	103
70	149	175	1670	110
80	160	187	1820	118
90	176	205	2020	130
95	191	224	2210	140

☐☐ ADA/ACC Cutpoints [1]

☐ AACC Cutpoints [2]

The medical decision cutpoints should be set so that the apoB and LDL-P cutpoints are equivalent to those for LDL-C in terms of population percentiles.

[1] Brunzell, et al. Diabetes Care 2008;31(4):811-822.
[2] Contois JH, et al. Clinical Chemistry 2009; 55:407-419

Goals

I think most doctors will try to get a patient's LDL-C to 100 if at medium risk and LDL-C to 70 if at high risk. They determine risk by gestalt. They don't use the Framingham score, and like the Ten Commandments, they probably can't name the five *major* risk factors exactly. I know this because I do get the Framingham score on most of my patients, and I have to check the details of the major risk factors often when I am with a patient. Even Dr. Bonow got it wrong in his conclusion in the September 2009 issue of *NEJM*. He wrote the case patient was low risk when he was actually intermediate risk. If the *NEJM* can get confused after deliberate thought and review, how can the family practitioner do it? I asked a young cardiologist if he uses the Framingham score. He says he does it in his head. Gestalt. NCEP is asking the family doctor to follow these very complicated guidelines, yet many professors feel the family doctor can't understand LDL particle number. They advise several different goals for LDL based on risk. No one follows it. Doctors will either treat to 100 LDL-C or 70 LDL-C. Most ignore the 130 LDL-C goal. NCEP then states if TGs are more than 200, the primary care doctor should get the non-HDL cholesterol to a goal thirty points higher than the LDL goal. This has been in place since 2001. Similar to the Framingham risk, I don't know any doctors in Topeka who do non-HDL goal.

KUMC professor Dr. Moriarty predicted that the new NCEP guidelines will replace LDL-C guidelines with non-HDL-C guidelines as the primary goal. I thought this was an astute prediction. It would be a compromise between the LDL particle number or APOB proponents and the LDL-C proponents.

My contribution is to change the name of non-HDL cholesterol to the Tubby Factor as 48% of patients with metabolic syndrome and large waists usually have discordance with their LDL-C. This means an LDL-C in these patients can be less than 70, as it was with Tim Russert, and yet have many other atherogenic particles that are not being measured. Tubby Factor immediately tells the patient this is a bad number, and losing weight is one way to get it lower. Every day I have to tell patients which is the good cholesterol and which is the bad cholesterol. The Tubby Factor by its name sounds bad.

The Tubby Factor or non-HDL cholesterol NCEP guideline goals are less than 100 in very high-risk patients and less than 130 in high-risk patients if their triglycerides are greater than 200.

The special report from *Clinical Chemistry* 55:3 by John Contois et al. states on page 415, "In terms of population equivalence to LDL-C goals, however, lower cutpoints appear more appropriate." They suggest less than 80 non-HDL-C for very high risk and less than 120 non-HDL-C for high risk. They do not go this far with LDL-P or APOB in table 5 on page 414.

At the Midwest National Lipid Association, Dr. Sniderman from Canada said he now believes the APOB goal for very high-risk patients is an APOB of less than 60.

I don't think it is a stretch to then make the LDL-P goal in very high-risk patients to be less than 750.

I have heard that this is too expensive. If it can be achieved with simvastatin and Endur-acin for less than $90 a year, I don't think that is true.

I have heard it is needlessly subjecting the patient to unneeded risk of the drugs. As long as you don't go above simvastatin 40 mg or Endur-acin 500 mg BID, I have found these drugs to be very safe.

If Zetia has to be added as a third drug, the argument of expense but not risk can be made. At that point, it is the physicians' job to determine with the patient what they want to do. Perhaps if the CAC is less than 25 or 100 and the CIMT percentile risk is less than 75 and the LDL-P is usually less than 1,000, judgment might call for not adding on the third drug to get to the goal of less than 750, especially if the patient has lost some weight and is exercising. If the next CIMT shows an increase in the wall thickness, I think the third drug should be added. If the CRPhs is high or the LpPLAC is high, that might make the push to the third drug.
HDL-C is not a goal of NCEP.
Triglycerides are not a goal of NCEP.
They are targets in patients with metabolic syndrome.

Targets, goals: pretty confusing.
I passed the lipidology boards, and I have to check the charts every day to make certain I have it right.

I have done hundreds of NMR LipoProfiles for LDL particle number paid for by Medicare. I often have found the non-HDL cholesterol(Tubby factor) to be normal but the LDL-P to be high. This is discordance. In the Offspring trial, LDL-P was more predictive than non-HDL cholesterol(Tubby factor) while non-HDL cholesterol was more predictive than LDL-C.

Many professors feel the LDL-P is too complicated for the average doctor. I disagree. Instead of worrying about two numbers(LDL-C and non-HDL-C),
LDL-P is just one number we need to get to goal.
What are the LDL-P goals?
Let us start with the ATP 2001 premise that a neutral LDL-C is 40.
Then look at the safety of getting patients to LDL-C 55 and some down to 35 in the JUPITER trial.

I use those two facts to practice a simple goal guideline.

LDL-P of less than 1,000 for high-risk patients
LDL-P of less than 750 for very high risk and/or to regress plaque

However, I think even low-risk patients may want to get their LDL-C to less than 100 or their LDL-P less than 1,000 with TLC, fish oil, and Endur-acin at an early age.

LDL-P of less than 750 is the second percentile of the human race.
Most professors would say that this goal is only for "the total vascular nightmares." This goal of less than 750, the professors would say "would bankrupt the USA for no good reason and it is subjecting patients to needless cost and side effects."

LDL-P of 1,000 to 1,100 is the 20th percentile where risk may begin.
Trouble really begins at an LDL-P greater than 1,300 to 1,400.

I don't think we will bankrupt the nation by ordering simvastatin and Endur-acin for less than $90 a year. I think aspirin is the most dangerous drug we give. If the patient is seen three times a year by a physician with lab work, the danger is minimal.

The physician is an important ingredient. Three visits a year is very important. This keeps the patient on track to goal and maintain goal.

—

The JUPITER trial is very important in this discussion. This is an outcome study in people choosing to start pharmacological prophylaxis. These patients had only one major risk factor—age. It was supposed to be a primary prevention study, as their LDL-Cs were in the normal range for their risk. However, it turns out that the APOB was 110 or the 70th percentile population cutpoint. Thus it turns out these were not low-risk people. Many of these people had metabolic syndrome. They are the Tubby people. They had the Tubby Factor.

Cardiovascular deaths and morbidity was on the down swing. However, because of the Tubby Factor, it is going back up (see Dayspring's reference in recent Lipoholics). America is getting tubby at a younger and younger age. Metabolic syndrome is seen in teenagers now. This may be the first generation that is buried by its parents because of heart disease. It is not enough to say lose weight and exercise when we have the tools to evaluate and treat in a safe, inexpensive way. The Philadelphia preventive heart center brochure allows any adult who is concerned to get a CAC. For anyone with the metabolic syndrome or family history, that is probably a good idea.

In 2003, after Prove-it and HPS, the NCEP updated its guidelines to allow physicians the option to get LDL-C to 70. It must be remembered that while the average LDL-C was 70 in the Prove-it trial, half of those patients were under 70. However, that message did not get to the physicians. If a patient is at LDL-C 75, the doctor will settle for it. Unfortunately, as I follow people every four months, I see that 75 go up to 95 during the holidays or due to poor compliance. The physicians need to try to get their patients under 70. If it is 50, don't decrease the statin, which is something I have seen physicians do.

When Medicare began paying for NMR LipoProfile three times a year, I began to order this test.
I am amazed at the amount of discordance between LDL-C and LDL-P. In very high-risk patients, I would have been happy with an LDL-C of 65, only to now see their LDL-P above 1,000 routinely. I have been adding on another drug rather than increasing the statin to maximum to get their LDL-P well below 1,000.

Many professors will say less than 750 LDL-P is too low because of expense and side effects. That has not been my experience. Expense is covered by simvastatin and Endur-acin, and side effects are less because I can afford to use a lower dose of the statin while adding Endur-acin. At 1,000 with Endur-acin, I have only had to stop approximately three patients because of flushing. No other serious side effects except perhaps one flare-up of gout.

It has been my experience in these very high-risk patients that one time I will find an LDL-P of 600, and four months later I will find an LDL-P of 800. I don't want to get them to LDL-P of 950 and then see them at 1,150 the next time. This is the clinical practice of medicine, and if I can give a patient two drugs without side effects or cost, I will aim for LDL-P of 750. As said before, the LDL-C neutral level as per ATP literature is 40, so I believe it is safe to get LDL-P very low. Babies make brains with LDL-Cs of 40. That is lipid-rich tissue.

I try to get my patients to an HDL-C of more than 50 by giving them Endur-acin. Exercise and weight loss in a Tubby patient can raise HDL-C 100% as it did for me. I don't try to push HDL-C above 60. If it's above 60, I don't worry about it. I like to see TGs less than 100.

Endur-acin raises HDL-C and lowers TGs. One thousand milligrams of Endur-acin is usually all you need to raise HDL-C. This is the safe dose as well. It may take a year to get to maximum levels of HDL-C.

Fish oil or more specifically omega-3 fatty acids called DHA and EPA will lower TG as well.
I try to get *all* patients on at least 850 mg of DHA plus EPA a day.
If TGs remain an issue, I advise Lovaza four tabs a day.

In the 4S trial in patients with a mean LDL-C 188 and a prior CHD event in an elderly group, there was a 98% absolute risk reduction with treatment.

This is what our goal should be. Let's prevent heart attacks and strokes. Let us start it early in the disease process. Identify who has vulnerable plaque and then treat them aggressively.

The JUPITER trial took patients that were theoretically healthy and reduced their risk with the highest dose of Crestor. Most of these patients did have the Tubby syndrome, and their average APOB was 110 or the 70th patient percentile.

In my practice, I am taking patients that have diseased arteries and the Tubby syndrome (metabolic syndrome) and taking them down to LDL-P of less than 750 or APOB of less than 60 or a Tubby Factor (non-HDL cholesterol) of less than 80.

I hope to stabilize the plaque I showed them to have and maybe even regress it. I hope there will be no sudden deaths in my population as a result. Why settle for anything less?

Chapter Nine

REGRESSION OF PLAQUE

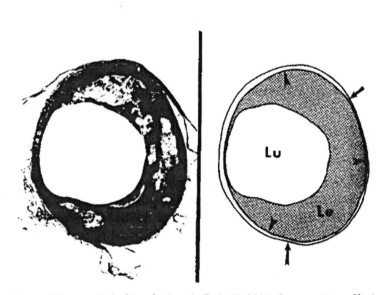

Figure 1. Photograph of a Cross Section of a Typical Left Main Coronary Artery with an Advanced Atherosclerotic Plaque (Left Panel), and a Corresponding Contour Tracing of the Artery (Right Panel).

The lumen (Lu) is clearly demarcated by the intimal surface. The internal elastic lamina (arrowheads) is readily discernible for most of the vessel circumference and almost always beneath the plaque as well, despite underlying atrophy of the media where the plaque and arterial wall tend to bulge outward (between the arrows). The area occupied by the lesion (Le) is shaded. The cross-sectional stenosis is defined as the extent to which the area encompassed by the internal elastic lamina — i.e., the potential lumen area if no plaque were present — is occupied by the lesion (percentage of stenosis = lesion area/internal elastic area × 100). In this vessel, the cross-sectional stenosis is 46 percent. Magnification, ×7.4.

The above photo is from the article "Compensatory Enlargement of Human Atherosclerotic Coronary Arteries" by Semour Glagov et al., *N Engl J Med*, 1987, 316:1371-5.

This is an important concept to understand: *plaque versus stenosis*.

The artery depicted above has a normal lumen, and there is plaque or atheroma in the wall of the artery. Dr. Glagov describes that plaque will fill in the wall and grow bigger, and the lumen size will be the same as before, and thus the angiogram (luminogram) will be normal. It's been well known that patients could have normal angiograms and then die the next day when their atheroma in the artery wall ruptured. The atheroma had not encroached on the lumen. Plaque was not seen on the angiogram.

What's very interesting is that once the plaque does get bigger and finally does encroach on the lumen of the artery, the stress test will still be normal despite obstruction of the lumen up to 70%. There needs to be 75% stenosis of an artery in the coronaries to have a positive nuclear stress test. However, sudden death often occurs with only 50% stenosis. A patient can have a normal stress test, and a month later the patient can die, as what happened with Tim Russert. The soft inflamed plaque ruptures, and this has to do with inflammation. This is why *C-reactive protein high sensitivity* or *LpLAC* levels are done to see how much inflammation the patient has.

The best test to show if you have any plaque in your heart is the *coronary artery calcium* (CAC) done with the CT scan, not the nuclear stress test or the coronary angiogram. A number is 1.0 or greater demonstrates that the patient has disease. Once diseased artery (plaque) is present, the plaque can become inflamed. With inflammation, the membrane of the plaque can rupture. Thrombosis develops over the site of the rupture, which will occlude the coronary artery and cause sudden death.

NCEP guidelines seem to state that the emerging risk factor of a coronary calcium score of more than 99 is a cardiac equivalent. The SHAPE trial states a calcium score of 1.0 or greater a positive test for atherosclerosis. I think if atherosclerosis is present, it is vulnerable to inflammation and may rupture, causing thrombosis and sudden death.

CIMT is an ultrasound of the intimal wall of the carotids. In many medical trials, it is used to demonstrate regression of plaque. The SHAPE trial considered a CIMT score of more than 49% to demonstrate presence of atherosclerosis. The SHAPE trial considers a CIMT of more than 74% or a carotid wall thickness of more than 0.99 mm to be a cardiac equivalent or high risk.

The Goals to obtain regression of atheroma

—LDL particle number < 750
—HDL-C > 50
—Triglycerides < 100
—Inflammation levels normal
—Blood pressure ≤130 systolic
—Waist 40 inches or less for men and less than 35 inches for women

The physician desk reference, PDR, presently states that niacin and colestipol together have the indication for regression of plaque. Colestipol is similar to the newer preparation Welchol. Crestor, and other statins, has the indication to slow progression; thus I advise using combination therapy to get to goals.

Meta-analysis review from *JAMA* (2/2007) titled "Post Hoc Analysis of 4 IVUS Trials," by Nichols, Nissan, et al., shows that 1,445 patients studied with IVUS with an LDL-C reduction from 124 to 87.5 and an increase of HDL by 7.5% had regression of plaque.

There is no evidence that regressing plaque improves outcome. Thus, it is not an NCEP ATP goal.

Lowering LDL-C has been shown to improve outcome. However, is it the LDL-C itself or the fact that as LDL-C goes down so does the inflammation of the artery?

You need about five thousand patients to demonstrate an improved outcome of survival. It took four studies just to get a total of 1,445 patients who had IVUS studies. It is very expensive to do intravenous ultrasound angiograms on patients. The ASTEROID trial 2006 used IVUS with 349 patients and showed regression on Crestor. There was not a statin-only arm? So FDA did not give Crestor the indication for regression of plaque. The LDL-C went down to 61 and increased HDL—C by 15% (43 to 49).

Before IVUS, QCA (quantitative coronary angiogram) was done in CLAS, FATS, and HATS. Two hundred patients was a big study. The problem with these studies is that an angiogram is a lumenogram. The QVC looks at the lumen, not the plaque that is in the wall of the artery.

It would be nice to do IVUS on five thousand patients and measure LDL-P, large and small HDL, and TG in head-to-head studies with statin plus different combination drugs. The drug companies don't like head-to-head studies ever since the *Prove-it* trial showed the competitors' drug to be more effective. However, it was still a smart move for pravastatin because it prevented people from bailing out on their drug as it was clear that Lipitor was much better at lowering LDL-C. Pravastatin salespeople said, "Wait till our study shows that pravastatin has a better outcome because it lowers inflammation better." After the study, it didn't matter because pravastatin came off patent.

Now we use CIMT to prove regression of plaque with drugs. This is an ultrasound of the carotid and not the coronaries. It deals in 1/1,000 of a millimeter change of atheroma. So far, only Crestor has received an indication for slowing progression of plaque by CIMT. They are trying to get the regression indication with more studies. The change in plaque size in the METEOR trial 3/2007 is so small. Placebo increased atheroma in carotid by 0.0131 mm.

Crestor 40 mg in low-risk group over twenty-four months decreased atheroma at twelve sites in the carotid measured by CIMT by 0.0014 mm. This was not significant enough to get the regression indication. LDL-C went from 155 to 78, and HDL went from 50 to 53 (8% increase).

Important question: What was the baseline CIMT?

Zetia was crucified because of its CASHMERE trial. The patients were not drug naive. They had a difficult disease called familial hypercholesterolemia. Their baseline CIMT was not that bad. It was a negative trial.
Later they had a better CIMT trial with the SANDS trial, but that has not restored their reputation.

Zetia company tells us to wait until 2012 for the completion of its *Improve-it trial*—eighteen thousand patients. It seems to be a similar strategy that pravastatin used. Keep using Zetia. You will see that it works in 2012.

Zetia is a great drug to reach goal of LDL-P less than 750. However, I will always try to use Endur-acin 500 mg BID and then add Zetia as a third drug.

Arbiter 6 trial just came out and showed niacin to be better than Zetia at regression in a head to head trial.

Chapter Ten

NEJM ARTICLE MISCALCULATES
THE FRAMINGHAM RISK SCORE

This is the case presented in the *New England Journal of Medicine* (NEJM) September 3, 2009.

Major Risk Factors
52-year-old male
Positive family history for CVD

First Mistake:

Framingham Score

Male 52 years old	6 points
Total cholesterol 220	3 points
Nonsmoker	0 points
HDL 38	2 points
BP 130 sys untreated	1 point
TOTAL	12 points

Ten-year risk is 10% or 1% per year.
The author states on page 995 the patient is at a low Framingham risk score.
He states the patient is a less than 10%.
In my calculation, the patient is at 10% or an intermediate risk.
This is the first mistake in the article.

Second Mistake
Let's say I am wrong. The patient is at low Framingham risk.
NCEP standards state initiate treatment if LDL-C is more than 160.
This patient is at 160. Thus, this author is not following the NCEP guidelines.

Third Mistake
Total cholesterol 220
minus HDL-C 38
Non-HDL cholesterol 182 (*Tubby Factor)*

If TG is more than 200, which I suspect it is, as HDL-C is less than 40:

NCEP non-HDL cholesterol goal (Tubby Factor) is less than 160, if he is trying to reach an LDL-C goal of less than 130 as per NCEP guideline for low-risk patients with LDL-C more than 160 after Rx with statin.

However, this patient is intermediate risk, and the treatment is initiated if LDL-C more than 130 and the LDC-C goal is less than 100 LDL with a non-HDL cholesterol (Tubby goal) goal of less than 130. It seems Dr. Bonow doesn't care about TG or non-HDL cholesterol (Tubby Factor) or APOB or LDL particle number.

This is why this patient needs a CAC. This *NEJM* doctor did use the guidelines correctly. We need to make it simple.

If CAC positive or CIMT positive, get LDL-P less than 1,000.

If you want to get regression of plaque, get LDL-P less than 750.

Dr. Bonow has a great list of references. However, let me add to them the following:

1. Falk, E., H. S. Hecht, M. Naghavi, et al. "From Vulnerable Plaque to Vulnerable Patient—Part III: Executive Summary of the Screening for Heart Attack Prevention and Education (SHAPE) Task Force Report." *Am J Cardiol.*; 98, suppl 2A (2006): 2H-15H.

"Recommends screening for subclinical atherosclerosis using computed tomography, carotid artery ultrasound, or both for all asymptomatic at risk' men aged 45-75 years and women aged 55-75."

"The SHAPE trial *considered a positive test for atherosclerosis*
   1.   a CACS of 1.0 or greater or
   2.   a CIMT greater than 49th percentile or
   3.   presence of carotid plaque."

"However, those considered high risk or CHD equivalent were further subcategorized as having a CAC > 100 or 75th percentile or CIMT > 0.99 mm or > 75th percentile."

This is my rationale for doing CIMT or CAC on cardiac equivalent patients or *diabetics*; what we call high-risk patients. I want to determine if they are very high risk. It affects what goals I treat patients to, something which Dr. Bonow does not discuss. High-risk patients should have NMR LipoProfiles done, and the LDL-P should at least be less than 1,000.
Very high-risk patients should have a LDL-P of less than 750.
I also try to treat high-risk patients with documented plaque to less than 750 to get regression of plaque. I try to document this with serial CIMTs every two years. I have demonstrated this on myself. Please see my YouTube site: bedwards1951.

The other references I use as a lipidologist are the following:

2. Sica, Dominic A. and Peter P. Toth. *Clinical Challenges in Lipid Disorders*. 2008. page 53, table 5.1 CHD equivalents summary.
3. Davidson, Michael H., Kevin Maki, and Peter Toth. *Therapeutics Lipidology*. 2007.
4. Blum, Conrad and Neil Stone. *Management of Lipids in Clinical Practice*. 6th ed. 2006.

Dr. Bonow writes on page 993, *NEJM*, September 3, 2009, "The identification of patients at increased risk is useful only if it leads to a successful strategy that helps avert future coronary events. No studies have been designed to demonstrate this effect."

We often don't practice solely on outcome studies.

Preventive medicine in particular depends much on the physician practicing medicine to the best of his ability and the resources available for an individual patient.

I researched some of the other screening tests.

Only two cancer screening tests meet the USPSTF criteria for a strong recommendation:

1. Pap smear
2. Fecal occult blood testing

These aim to remove precancerous lesion, prevent invasive cancer, save the involved organ, and reduce disease-specific mortality.

More controversial cancer screening tests:

1. PSA
2. Mammogram

These detect invasive cancers and lead to aggressive treatments.

In 2002, USPSTF included screening colonoscopy as an option, but with the qualification that the potential added benefits of colonoscopy may not always be great enough to justify the increased risks and inconvenience. Over five hundred patients have to be screened to prevent one invasive cancer.

In 2004, it was predicted 215,990 cases of invasive breast cancer would be diagnosed.

A Danish meta-analysis in 2000 concluded there was no evidence that mammography reduced mortality from breast cancer.

US investigators included more positive trials and had a positive result.

National Cancer Institute's Physician Data Query program largely endorsed the idea that most of the mammography trials were seriously flawed.

USPSTF demoted mammography from grade A to grade B.

One thousand two hundred women aged 40 to 70 years must be invited to be screened four to five times over ten years to prevent one death from breast cancer.

Women who get ten annual mammograms have a 50% chance that at least one of them is a false positive result. Many of these will get a biopsy.

This week, a panel advised that screening mammograms should start at age fifty because the evidence shows that too many false positives are found from 40 to 49 years of age. This leads to unnecessary biopsies. It leads to anxiety in patients. I suspect it does find cancer early in some individuals, but for society it is too expensive. This is an example of health care rationing.

I think many women will continue to get mammograms early but they will have to pay for it themselves. On *Morning Joe*, Mr. Scarborough complains that the richest nation on earth should be able to pay to prevent breast cancer in the 1/2,000 mammograms that the early screening provides. Minutes before he was complaining about the federal deficit. This does not compute. We need to cut back somewhere, and this scientific statement is showing us how to cut back. I might suggest we take the money from the military industrial complex and start a preventive health complex instead. I think CAC/CIMT will save money in the long run to prevent hospitalizations and angiograms and nuclear stress tests. It's not clear to me why we are in Germany, Korea, Iraq, and Afganistan. It seems leaving those places would pay for a comprehensive health program. What is clear to me is that rationing of health services is already here. Mostly, the private insurance companies are the ones that make the patient take the generic version of the statins. There is no generic for Zetia, and yet they take patients off that drug as well. I believe cancer of the colon can be seen as early as age 35, and yet the screening colonoscopy is begun at age 50. Physicians have the greatest longevity among the professions because of access to health care. I had my first sigmoidoscopy at age 35 and my first colonoscopy at age 40. I knew it was a cancer that could be prevented if found early, so why not check? Last year, I had my first colon polyp found.

Criteria for Evaluating a Screening Program

1. Does the program target a disease that causes serious morbidity and mortality that might be prevented by the service?
2. Can the screening test accurately identify healthy people who are at high risk for developing advanced disease?
3. Does treatment given before symptoms occur result in better outcomes that treatment given later?
4. Is the screening test feasible to use in primary care?
5. Do the overall benefits outweigh the harms of screening and treatment?

Source: ACP medicine text, p. 40.

My Opinion

1. Does the program target a disease that causes serious morbidity and mortality that might be prevented by the service?

As Dr. Bonow writes on page 990, "Cardiovascular disease remains the leading cause of death in developed countries as well as in most developing countries and there is a concern that the growing prevalence of obesity and type 2 Diabetes will reverse the gains of the past 40 years."

I think it is much easier to treat subclinical atherosclerosis at an earlier age. Just my opinion, it will prevent clinical atherosclerosis. There are many primary preventive studies such as JUPITER trial that had a positive outcome.

2.   Can the screening test accurately identify healthy people who are at high risk for developing advanced disease?

Yes. Positive CAC or CIMT increases a patients risk profile as per NCEP. Framingham low-risk persons will become high risk if they have a CAC of more than 100.

3.   Does treatment given before symptoms occur result in better outcomes than treatment given later?

I need help with this one.

NNTT 4S trial for all CAD deaths, major CAD event = ten (secondary prevention)

NNTT CARE trial for all fatal and nonfatal CAD events = thirty-three (secondary prevention)

NNTT VA-HIT for fatal and nonfatal CAD events = three (secondary prevention)

NNTT WOSCOPS for first fatal and nonfatal CAD events = forty-eight (primary prevention)

NNTT TexCaps for risk of first major CAD event = fifty-eight (primary prevention)

Treatment works better in sicker patients?

But compare these numbers to mammography and colonoscopy. You have to treat thirty breast cancer patients to prevent one death with chemo, radiation, and surgery. A forty-year-old woman has 1.47% chance (1/68) of developing breast cancer within ten years.

4. Is the screening test feasible to use in primary care?

We have CAC and CIMT in the great city of Topeka. Cost is $300 for CAC and $100 for CIMT.

Mammogram costs? Colonoscopy costs? CAC for $200 is available in Lawrence.

5. Do the overall benefits outweigh the harms of screening and treatment?

In my opinion, the way to prevent clinical atherosclerosis is to treat subclinical atherosclerosis. Then there will be less nuclear stress tests, angioplasties with stents, and surgery. One CAC is equal to three CXRs in terms of radiation exposure.

CIMT is ultrasound, and we can do it every two years to determine effectiveness of treatment. If disease progresses despite good patient compliance and having a LDL-P of 750, HDL-C of more than 50, and TG of less than 100 maybe we should then get a 128-slice angio CT of the coronaries to see what is going on.

This is the screening plan I would like to see us institute in Topeka.

Yes, the benefit does outweigh the harm.

Moderate-dose statin plus Endur-acin 1,000 mg plus fish oil is very safe especially if monitored by a physician.

Dr. Bonow writes on page 992, "It remains unclear whether CAC scanning has a favorable effect on clinical outcomes."

Then on page 993, "The major unresolved question is whether routine, widespread CAC screening or determination of the CAC score in an individual patient will lead to an overall improvement in quality of care and clinical outcomes. The identification of patients at increased risk is useful only if it leads to a successful strategy that helps avert future coronary events. Since no studies have been designed to demonstrate this effect, there are no convincing data to suggest that this desired result can be achieved."

In response to this paragram, I will quote a paragraph from an interview of the inventor of the calcium score, Dr. Agatston:

Everyday Health: There is some controversy about the usefulness of the calcium score. Why?

Dr. Agatston: The naysayers complain that there is no evidence from randomized clinical trials that noninvasive screening for hidden disease will ultimately reduce the number of heart attacks. This criticism ignores the fact that to perform such a clinical trial would mean withholding preventive treatment to many participating patients who were found to have high calcium scores. Doing so would simply be unethical, given the totality of evidence demonstrating the risk of having accumulated significant coronary calcium. In fact, no informed patient would give their consent to enroll in such a study.

My clinical experience leaves no question that CAC has a favorable effect on clinical outcomes.

It is the poker-hand analogy. With risk factors, I can only guess what cards are in my patient's hands. I really don't know his disease state.

With CIMT and CAC, I can see the poker hand that my patient has. I don't have to guess.

When betting on life and death, I want to see that poker hand. I want to know if my patient has subclinical atherosclerosis that is vulnerable to inflammation and may rupture, causing one of the 100,000 sudden deaths a year, many of which the first symptom of disease is sudden death.

On a daily basis, I discover disease, and I change the aggressiveness of my treatment accordingly. Many of my patients will pay $100 cash to get CIMT.

Many of our young people are becoming overweight at an early age. We need to find subclinical atherosclerosis and treat them early.

The presence of plaque in the coronaries and/or the carotids plus the metabolic syndrome elevates a patient from high risk to very high risk for a cardiac event.

I have found this in many of my patients. You will find it also if you start looking. Treat their LDL-P to at least less than 1,000 or better yet less than 750. Moderate dose of a statin with Endur-acin will get you there with minimal side effects.

Check the vitamin-D level to avoid muscle pain.

Dr. Bonow writes on page 994, "Two observational studies reported that knowledge of a positive CAC scan was associated with greater use of statin and Aspirin therapy and risk-reducing changes in lifestyle." He also quotes a randomized trial that did not show any difference.

This is where I have to rely on my experience. Selling statins has been a hard sell. Selling exercise and diet is still an almost impossible sell.

I am asking a patient who feels well to take a medicine that often feels to him to be causing his muscle pain.

Once I teach him about vulnerable plaque and inflammation causing rupture of plaque and then I show him he has plaque with two very sensitive methods of imaging (CIMT and CAC), I now have his attention.

The NCEP guidelines are outdated in terms of treatment goals.

Clearly, the JUPITER trial showed that LDL-C as low as 35 is safe.

The normal LDL-C may be 40, as babies do well with this level.

Thus, I am very aggressive in my goals.

For a patient with high risk, I will try to get their LDL-P to less than 1,000.

For a patient with plaque, I will try to get their LDL-P to less than 750 to get regression of plaque.

I advise doing the CIMT every two years to monitor progress.

I check the LDL-P every four months. Medicare pays for this.

It is only by following a patient closely and showing them progress with imaging and with goals that we can hope to have a patient compliant with taking his medicine.

Chapter Eleven

CORONARY ARTERY CALCIUM

In the summary and final conclusions on page 396 in the *JACC* volume 49, number 3 by Greenland et al. (2007), the ACCF/AHA Expert Consensus Document of Coronary Artery Calcium Scoring states *it may be reasonable to consider use of CAC measurement in asymptomatic patients with intermediate CHD risk (between 10-20% ten-year risk of estimated coronary events)*.

I have a problem with this advice. The Framingham risk score and the ATP-II call HDL-C of more than 60 a negative risk factor. Many studies have shown very high HDL-C to be associated with risk. HDL-C of less than 40 is considered a major risk factor. On individual patients, these two guidelines may be perfectly wrong. Plasma HDL-C is the least accurate of standard lipid measurements. Performed correctly, HDL-C accuracy is more or less 10%. That means my patient comes in with an HDL-C of 39; he may actually have an HDL-C of 43 and thus not have a major risk factor. This is why I think getting a CAC and a CIMT is the best way to show the doctor and the patient that the patient is at high risk. Once a plaque is shown to be present, there is a risk inflammation will cause it to rupture.

Seymour Glagov, MD, published an article titled "Compensatory Enlargement of Human Atherosclerotic Coronary Arteries" in the *New England Journal of Medicine* (1987, 316:1371-5). He states that "lumen stenosis is delayed until the lesion occupies approximately 40% of the potential lumen area." This explained why a patient with a normal coronary angiogram might die the next day with a ruptured plaque. It also explains why Tim Russert died one month after a normal nuclear stress test. There has to be more than 75% stenosis of the lumen of the artery before the nuclear stress test will be positive. A person with a negative stress test may have a great deal of plaque that is vulnerable to inflammation and rupture. When that membrane of the plaque ruptures, it can occlude the artery, cutting off blood supply to that part of the heart. That causes a heart attack and possibly ventricular fibrillation which causes sudden death.

CAC CT scan is the most sensitive test for coronary artery disease. Its biggest disadvantage is the radiation. It also is not advised for showing regression of plaque although there are stories of regression including my personal history. I think CAC is the best way to discover subclinical atherosclerosis in patients with at least one risk factor for heart disease. This means every man more than forty-four years old and every woman more than fifty-four years old. If mammography screening is worthwhile, I believe CAC screening is reasonable.

Once he has a calcium score of one or greater, the patient knows he has plaque. Under the SHAPE trial, the patient has atherosclerosis. Under the NCEP guidelines, the calcium score needs to be more than 99 to be a cardiac equivalent.

I worry that once plaque is demonstrated, it is vulnerable to inflammation and subsequent rupture. Often in young patients, the soft plaque has not been calcified, and thus the calcium score underestimates the true plaque burden. Often in patients less than sixty years old, the calcium score is zero, but the CIMT shows a more than 25% risk for an event. I believe these are high-risk patients and should have their LDL-P less than 1,000, and if it is not too difficult, it is reasonable to shoot for less than 750 to try for regression of plaque. This regression of atheroma can be documented in serial CIMTs. If Tim Russert had serial CIMTs, he would not have been reassured by a negative nuclear stress one month before he died. If we treat CACs of 1 or more to LDL-P of less than 750, we will decrease the 100,000 sudden deaths in this country. The first symptom of cardiac sudden death is often the event of sudden death. With CAC and CIMT, we have the tools to find these patients and prevent progression of plaque, if not regression of plaque.

The argument of cost is spurious. I have many patients on simvastatin and Endur-acin for less that $90 a year. If cost is an issue, then don't add Zetia and settle for a LDL-P less than 1,000. I worry that many patients who are treated to LDL-P of less than 1,000 are often above 1,000. If the goal is less than 750 and they forget pills sometimes, they will always be under LDL-P of less than 1,000.

I think the JUPITER trial shows that there is benefit with lower LDL-C and that it is safe. It is time to get aggressive.

CACs of more than 300 were associated with a 6.7% absolute risk of CHD as compared to those with CACS 0 (0.3%) (Laboski, S. G. et al. 2007, *Arch Intern Med*, 167 (22):2437-2442).

Chapter Twelve

CIMT IS NOT A DUPLEX CAROTID ULTRASOUND

The *Tubby plan* calls for getting a CIMT and a CAC on patients to determine if the patient has subclinical atherosclerosis. CAC may miss the soft plaque in younger patients that have not had time for calcium to appear in the plaque. The CIMT complements the CAC in picking up plaque in the carotids. Usually if there is plaque in the carotids, there is also plaque in the coronaries.

In the chart below, I had eleven patients in my practice that had a zero CAC or calcium score. They thought they were bulletproof. They were ready to go off their diets and throw away their pills. I convinced them to get a CIMT, and we showed them that they were at more than 75% more risk for a cardiac event than another person their age. This puzzle is explained by the fact that younger patients less than sixty often have soft coronary plaque or atheroma that has not yet been calcified.

I became certified in osteoporosis. I did this so I could qualify to read DEXA scans at my hospital. Medicare allows us to do these scans every two years to determine if a patient develops osteoporosis or osteopenia. It is also used to monitor if a patient's bisphosphonate (Fosamax, Actonel, or Boniva) is working. The scan subjects the patient to a small amount of radiation and is very technician dependent in terms of accuracy. Repeat scans should be done on the same machine, and the machine should be calibrated frequently. If the patient is not in the same exact position as the last DEXA scan, it is not as reliable.

Age	sex	DM	Met Syn	CAC	CIMT	cimt%	Carotid Stenosis	LDLp	non-HDL	LDLc	HDL	TG	Total CHOL	Statin	Enduracin	Zetia
64	M	Y		+CATH	1.05	>75	9	716	85	59	68	130	153	C20		Y
73	M			+CATH	0.97	>75		1313	121	87	31	170	152			
77	M			+CATH	0.95	>75		1145	85	56	52	143	137	S40	Y	Y
44	M			+CATH	0.91	>75		1197	89	57	46	158	135	C20	Y	Y
69	M			220	1.14	>75		1201	120	95	59	127	179			
81	F			110	1.06	>75		845	46	33	52	65	98	C10		Y
62	M			97	0.9	>75		958	63	50	43	67	106	C20	Y	Y
59	F			73	0.87	>75		639	83	71	74	59	157	C5		
71	F			66	1.06	>75		1422	99	59	32	200	131	C5	Y	
53	M		3	48	0.81	>75		1012	70	61	51	44	121	C20	Y	
55	M		3	28	1.2	>75		1011	94	138	44	62	138	S10	Y	
55	F		5	1	0.85	>75		937	59	40	67	95	126	S40		Y
47	M		3	1	0.76	>75		762	62	51	46	54	108	L40	Y	
58	M			0	1.17	>75		1336	135	117	46	90	181	S40		
77	F			0	1.04	>75		2141	160	140	50	100	210		Y	
57	M			0	0.99	>75		439	77	39	61	191	138	C10	Y	
73	F			0	0.99	>75		838	78	67	81	57	159		Y	Y
65	F		5	0	0.9	>75		977	102	80	57	108	159	L40		
56	F		1	0	0.81	>75		769	77	64	86	63	163	S20		
54	M			0	0.76	>75		1220	109	82	54	133	163	C10		Y
57	F		3	0	0.76	>75				192	53	231		C5/O		
48	F			0	0.7	>75		758	90	77	84	65	174	C5		
79	F		4		1.06	>75		966	80	50	49	151	129	C10	Y	
70	F	Y			1.05	>75		1063	84	61	58	116	142	C40		Y
59	M		3		0.91	>75		1398	118	92	46	131	164	C10	Y	
58	M			0	0.79	74		1253	104	94	46	50	150	C5		
75	M		3	+CATH	0.92	70	20	469	65	54	65	53	130	S20		
65	M				0.69	59		1041	80	68	57	60	137	L40		
69	M			POS	0.79	50		598	66	53	54	64	120	C5	N1000	
54	M			+cath	0.72	50		355	254	50	24	2674	278			
60	M	Y	5	+CATH	0.71	50		1221	107	77	44	149	151	C5	Y	
65	F			+CATH	0.65	50		708	91	79	65	60	156		Y	
71	M			+ CATH	0.88	50		1233	106	67	42	195	148	S20		Y
75	M			+ CATH	0.88	50		830	77	57	63	98	140	S80		Y

69	F		5	+ CATH	0.77	50	9	1098	61	47	61	70	122	S40	Y	Y
71	M			566	0.74	50		1017	96	79	58	87	154	C40	Y	Y
58	M			370	0.71	50		1074	96	73	65	113	161	C20		
68	M			141	0.77	50		1242	115	99	61	80	176			
61	M		4	118	0.63	50		1636	111	90	42	105	153	C10	Y	
61	M		4	104	0.74	50		1192	99	76	44	114	143	L20	Y	
69	F	Y	4	70	0.85	50		1510	115	85	67	149	182	C5/O		
40	M			40	0.6	50		1225	185	0	0	0	185			
84	F		4	33	0.83	50		509	81	65	91	78	172	L20	Y	
57	M			28		50		713	72	60	55	60	127	C5		
57	F		4	26	0.62	50		854	73	44	57	143	130	C10		
73	M			20	0.72	50	39	678	68	57	57	56	125	C5	Y	
60	M		2	19	0.78	50		1399	88	78	56	50	144	S40	Y	
69	M			11	0.68	50		593	53	43	76	49	129	S10		
71	F		3	5.5	0.74	50		1228	110	102	73	41	183			
71	F		3	5.5	0.74	50		1029	93	79	68	68	161			
71	F		3	5.5	0.74	50		1194	80	71	74	43	154	C10		Y
61	M		3	3	0.62	50		958	63	56	60	35	123	S40	Y	Y
68	M		2	0.1	0.72	50	NOR-MAL	813	65	46	69	97	134	S40		
61	M		3	0	0.84	50	-	1315	109	87	44	82	153	C5		
60	M		1	0	0.78	50			146	116	59	129	205		Y	
80	M		2	0	0.78	50		718	106	93	59	67	165	LES80		
55	M			0	0.72	50	9		78	67	50	55	128	C10		
69	F			0	0.71	50	39	1104	84	68	58	78	142	C10	Y	
71	M			0	0.69	50		914	84	58	36	131	120	S10		Y
58	M			0	0.66	50		1094	129	111	54	91	183	S20		
55	F		2	0	0.64	50		1186	113	102	52	57	165			
48	M		3	0	0.63	50		2007	133	111	40	108	173			
56	M			0	0.63	50		1511	126	100	42	130	168	S5		
55	F			0	0.62	50		663	81	72	73	44	154			
49	F			0	0.62	50		1439	129	110	41	95	170			
55	F			0	0.61	50		923	98	84	71	68	169	C5		
57	M		3	0	0.61	50		1072	89	77	50	61	139	C20		
39	M		4	0	0.58	50		1088	124	100	51	120	175	C10	Y	
47	M		3	0	0.58	50		825	89	34	41	275	130		Y	
46	M			0	0.57	50		1368	156	132	49	121	205			
39	M		3	0	0.54	50		1433	134	102	39	159	173	C5	Y	
74	F				0.87	50		832	100	87	86	67	186	S10		
65	F				0.84	50		1938	164	115	53	247	217		Y	
65	F		5		0.83	50		1062	91	76	84	74	175	L10		
73	F		2		0.78	50		751	85	72	75	63	160	C5/O		
72	F	Y			0.77	50		761	80	34	46	232	126	C10		

57	F				0.76	**50**				92	66	80		C10	Y	
78	F				0.75	**50**		905	53	36	64	85	117	C20		Y
57	M				0.72	**50**		686	77	32	86	225	163	C5		
67	F		3		0.7	**50**	NOR-MAL	2398	230	185	61	226	291			
72	F		2		0.7	**50**		1843		149	42	239				
73	F				0.69	**50**		894	95	82	65	63	160	S10		
53	F				0.67	**50**		2249	171	147	55	156	226			
51	F	Y	5		0.67	**50**			188	132	43	278	231			
48	F		3		0.63	**50**		1485	127	104	53	116	180	S10		
56	F				0.61	**50**		940	82	71	69	53	151	L40		
57	F		3		0.6	**50**		1122	117	103	92	69	209	C10		
58	M		1		0.6	**50**		840	76	68	52	40	128	C10		
38	M				0.59	**50**				123	38			C40	Y	
50	F	Y	5		0.55	**50**		681	107	71	53	180	160	S40		
48	F	Y			0.54	**50**		381	60	39	71	107	131	C5		
69	F		2	+CATH	0.64	**<25**		1388	175	149	70	131	245	C5/O	Y	
62	F			+CATH	0.57	**<25**				107	59			L10	Y	
55	M			+CATH	0.56	**<25**		1107	81	69	38	60	119	S80	Y	Y
58	M		5	+CATH	0.55	**<25**	9	1057	131	96	50	173	181	C10	Y	
65	M			+CATH	0.62	**<25**	NOR-MAL	1055	61	53	58	40	119	S80	Y	Y
52	M			3871	0.57	**<25**		401	68	46	98	111	166	C5		
80	F			1434	0.71	**<25**		1021	158	143	64	77	222		Y	
70	F			199	0.69	**<25**		885	66	57	77	43	143	LES80		Y
70	M			186	0.54	**<25**		622	64	43	33	105	97	C5	Y	
53	M		5	57	0.53	**<25**		775	83	57	37	129	120	C10		Y
73	M	Y		25	0.56	**<25**		975	89	80	76	46	165	C10		
69	M		2	17	0.58	**<25**	9	970	51	45	64	31	115	C40	Y	Y
60	M			12	0.54	**<25**		1322	135	101	52	169	187	L40		Y
80	F		4	6	0.68	**<25**		626	59	29	51	148	110	S20		
58	M			5	0.54	**<25**		791	78	67	78	53	156	S40		Y
67	M		4	2	0.67	**<25**		605	73	55	68	88	141	C20	Y	
71	F		2	0	0.62	**<25**		732	82	70	76	61	158	P40	Y	
54	M			0	0.58	**<25**		676	66	46	44	100	110	L10	Y	
62	F		3	0	0.56	**<25**		926	79	70	65	43	144	C5		
61	M		0	0	0.54	**<25**	NOR-MAL	1028	149	129	67	99	216		Y	
67	F				0.66	**<25**	9	668	88	72	77	79	165			
71	F				0.61	**<25**	+	836	104	93	82	56	186	C5/O		
56	M				0.6	**<25**		829	80	71	43	44	123	L40	Y	
65	F				0.55	**<25**		781	121	113	92	40	213	C5		
57	F		4		0.53	**<25**			96	77	53	93	149	S40		Y

25	M				0.49	<25		999	117	82	71	176	188			
47	F		2		0.49	<25				68	70	74		C10		
46	M		4		0.48	<25		848	83	66	34	86	117	C5	Y	
44	F		4		0.46	<25				96	38	461		S20		Y
49	M		3		0.44	<25			145	116	41	145	186	S20		
82	M			+cath	0.89			1091	53	40	40	64	93	C40	Y	Y
56	F			0	0.88			1388	109	95	108	72	217	C5		
59	M			124	0.83			1039	70	60	46	51	116	C20		
63	M			88	0.62			754	85	71	69	68	154	C10		
53	F		3	0	0.59			1269	140	121	63	97	203	C20	Y	Y

The main argument against using CIMTs in clinical practice is the accuracy. The investigational studies such as METEOR had differences in the thousands to make the study significant. My CIMT reports come back in the hundredths, and it is a semiautomated machine looking at one area. I have been told it is more reliable than the older manual method. The people who do my scans are trained professionals doing other ultrasound scans. I think the quality is as good as or better than the average DEXA scan that Medicare pays for.

CIMTs, unlike DEXA scans, have no radiation. In Topeka, the CIMT costs $100.

This is a great tool to find hidden atheroma and patients at risk for rupture of plaque.

The above report shows eleven CACs that were zero. These patients thought they were bulletproof. I did the CIMT only to find they had a greater than 75th percentile risk for a cardiac event. These patients were very grateful and more motivated to do their TLC (exercise and diet). Seven of those patients were under sixty years old, and one was under fifty.

A CIMT with a thickness of more than 1.00 mm or more than 75th percentile is considered an emerging CHD equivalent (*Clinical Challenges in Lipid Disorders*, p. 53).

The SHAPE task force considered a CIMT of more than 49th percentile or the presence of carotid plaque on duplex carotid ultrasound as a positive test for atherosclerosis.

The SHAPE statement makes more sense to me if we are looking for vulnerable plaque that might rupture and cause sudden death or stroke.

I have eighteen patients that had CAC zero but a CIMT at 50% range. Thirteen of these patients were younger than sixty years old. Of these thirteen, four were under fifty and two were under forty.

Since January 2009, I have found twenty-nine patients with hidden plaque risk by the help of a CIMT for only $100.

In terms of statistics, it may be insignificant, but for patients in my practice, it is very significant. It does not lead to further invasive testing. It prevents nuclear stress tests and angioplasties as we start treatment at an early age to an aggressive goal of LDL-P less than 750 with a therapy that may cost only $90 a year (simvastatin and Endur-acin).

The sixth edition of *Management of Lipids in Clinical Practice* by Stone and Blum states on page 216 the following clinical tip: "Non-invasive imaging of the carotid arteries is a potential tool for following the results of lipid therapy. In MARS, for every 0.03 mm increase per year in carotid IMT, there was a significant increase in the relative risk for both fatal and nonfatal MI and for any coronary event" (Hodis et al. 1998).

Chapter Thirteen

LDL-P

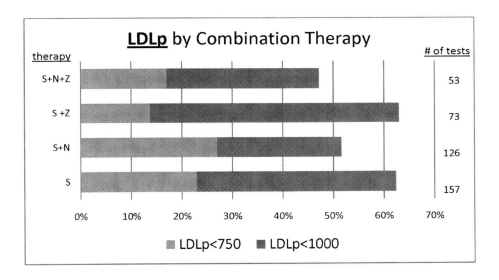

The patient spreadsheet illustrates two points here.

1. **Don't decrease therapy if LDL-C is less than 60; follow LDL-P**. I have twenty-six patients whose LDL-P is less than 750, and their LDL-C is between 39 and 35. JUPITER trial often had patients' LDL-C down to 35 without ill effect. I have thirty patients whose LDL-C is less than 35 but whose LDL-P is at goal at less than 750. I don't know of any studies about patients in this range of LDL-C. I just think it is not relevant. (Visit Dr. Dayspring's Lipidaholic blog on October 5, 2008. He presents a patient that requires more therapy with an LDL-C of 38.) Of these patients with very low LDL-C, only two are on maximum-dose statin.

Lipitor 80 mg was safe in the TNT trial, and Crestor 40 mg was safe in the JUPITER trial.

2. **Don't increase therapy if LDL-C is more than 70 if already at LDL-P goal.** I have fifty-five patients with LDL-C of more than 70. Many aggressive physicians might increase their medication. However, more medication is not needed as these patients have LDL-P less than 750. They are already to goal.

It's not the LDL-C, it's the LDL-P. The above is what *LDL-C discordance with LDL-P* is all about. It makes a difference in therapeutic decisions.

Once Medicare began paying for NMR Liposcience Lipoprofile, I began to realize how often I was treating patients incorrectly with the routine lipid panel.

The problem with traditional cardiovascular risk factor assessment is that they accurately predict risk in populations of patients but may not be adequate when applied to individual patients.

I can only suggest to other physicians to start ordering NMR LDL-P particle numbers or APOBs. The physicians will immediately see changes they will need to make in the therapy of their patients.

Dr. H. Robert Superko writes in *Circulation* May 5, 2009 on page 2383, "Advanced lipoprotein tests lend insight into subtle yet important aspects of lipoproteins and atherosclerosis that help to explain the relative failure of the LDL-C lowering strategy to stem the epidemic of atherosclerosis."

I get my LDL-P from NMR LipoScience LipoProfile. NMR stands for nuclear magnetic resonance. This is a mass spectrometer. The NMR measures the terminal methyl groups in the lipid within the particle. The amplitude of the methyl NMR signal is higher as the number of methyl groups goes up. The amplitude signal serves as the concentration of the lipoprotein.

Size doesn't matter? If the LDL-P is treated to goal, I don't worry about the size of the LDL-P. In the *Annals of Internal Medicine* (150:474-484), a systematic review was published in April 2009. On page 482, it states, "The studies generally found that LDL particle number (an NMR measurement) was associated with incident cardiovascular disease, but LDL particle size and small LDL particle fraction were not as consistently associated with incident disease."

Chapter Fourteen

THE TRUTH ABOUT HDL-C?

The highest HDL-C in my spreadsheet is HDL-C 111. The HDL-P was 30.
The lowest HDL-C was 28. The HDL-P was 27.
Which one has the better HDL?

HDL-C is a conundrum. Too little is no good, and many times too much is no good.
We are not certain which is better: the large HDL-P or the small HDL-P.

On page 37 of the 2009 text *Therapeutic Strategies in Lipid Disorders* by
Tonkin, it states, "There is overwhelming epidemiological evidence of an
inverse relationship between the risk of cardiovascular events and the plasma
concentration of HDL-C." That's great, but what should I do in my practice?

In *JAMA* 2007 (298[7]:786-798), the lead author Inder M. Singh states, "The
simple goal of increasing levels of 'good' cholesterol can no longer be applied
to all forms of HDL without consideration of therapeutic effect on HDL function
and ultimately cardiovascular risk."

Here is the best truth for today that I can discern from the article below.

1. Increase the HDL-C from 20 to 40 mg/dl and you get a large increase
    in total HDL-P.
2. Once the HDL-C goes above 40-45 mg/dl, there is little increase in
    HDL-P. Instead, the small HDL-P will fill up with cholesterol and become
    large HDL-P.

The Tubby guidelines try to get the patient's HDL-C to more than 50. That is
not the critical number. If the LDL-P is less than 750, I don't think the physician
needs to worry too much about the TG or the HDL-C.

After you get the LDL-P to goal, you can add the HDL-P (small, medium, and large sizes) on the second page of the NMR report to see where the HDL-P is in relation to HDL-C. The new NMR report adds up the total HDL-P. It may help you make some decisions in therapy, but I would not add niacin to Trilipex to Actos washed down with a glass of red wine to raise the HDL-P. Instead, encourage the patient to lose weight and exercise an hour a day.

Niacin raises the large HDL-P while Trilipex raises the small HDL-P. Both drugs improve the HDL-P functionality.

Someday we will be able to test the functionality in Topeka and clear up the confusion. Jacques Genest in *JACC* (200:51:643-644) states, "Given the multiple potentially beneficial effects of HDL on cardiovascular biology, there is scientific support for the concept that raising small HDL particles (often referred to as 'nascent' HDL particles) may be more important than generating large, cholesterol-rich HDL particles. Drugs that modulate HDL-C levels can be conceptually seen as those that decrease catabolism (CETP inhibitors, possibly niacin) and those that increase the production rate (fibrates . . . "

Inder M. Singh et al. in *JAMA* 2007 state, "The functionality of different HDL subfractions appears to vary substantially. Of the known forms of HDL-C (pre-B HDL, HDL2, HDL3) pre-B HDL appears to be the most anti-atherogenic form."

I think the best statement about HDL-C comes from Dr. William Cromwell in his paper, "High-Density Lipoprotein Associations with Coronary Heart Disease: Does Measurement of Cholesterol Content Give the Best Result?" *Journal of Clinical Lipidology* (2007, 1,57-64).

Dr. Cromwell states, "Although HDL-C is thought to indicate the quantity of circulating HDL particles, it is under appreciated that the amount of cholesterol carried inside lipoprotein particles is highly variable among individuals with the same HDL-C. Collectively, the data leads to the conclusion that both large and small HDL subclasses are cardioprotective."

Dr. Dayspring has taught me what I know about HDL-C/HDL-P in the following Lipidaholics blogs:

December 4, 2008

May 13, 2009
May 25, 2009

HDLp	Large HDL-P	Medium HDL-P	Small HDL-P
53.7	17.5	0.4	35.8
30.9	19.5	0.0	11.4
43.4	19.3	0.2	23.9
54.2	16.9	11.4	25.9
51.8	18.7	5.5	27.6
32.7	19.3	0.4	13.0
31.6	20.8	0.0	10.8
31.0	12.1	9.0	9.9

I called LipoScience to find out what the normal HDL-P amounts are, and they gave me this ballpark answer:

HDL-P sum: 35.1

	Large HDL-P	Medium HDL-P	Small HDL-P
75th percentile	9	7	22
50th percentile	6	3-4	19
25th percentile	3-4	1.0	16

NMR LipoScience does not measure the pre-B HDL.

Chapter Fifteen

THE LIPID PANEL/LIPOPROFILE

What is normal LDL-C? Is it 40 to 50?

LDL-C more than 100 is atherogenic.

LDL-C less than 70 is the 2% level for the population as per Framingham Offspring study.

JUPITER trial took normal patients to LDL-C average of 55 (as low as 35) with positive outcome results.

Complex hypobetalipoproteinemic patients have congenital low LDL-C less than 40 and live to their nineties.

If the non-HDL cholesterol is normal, then it doesn't matter what the LDL-C is, see *Am J Cardiol* (2006, 98:1363-1368) by NCEP chairman Scott Grundy.

Age	sex	DM	Met Syn	CAC	CIMT	cimt%	Carotid Stenosis	LDLp	NON-HDL	LDLc	HDL	TG	Total CHOL	Statin	Enduracin	Zetia	WelTri
75	F							3039	314	237	38	384	352				
53	F				0.67	50		2249	171	147	55	156	226				
76	F			+CATH			59	1656	331	N/C	53	435	384				WEL
75	F							3125	269	198	55	363	324				
75	F							2245	233	181	68	258	301				
68								2473	185	136	84	245	269				
62	M							2135	195	120	61	375	256				
48	M		3	0	0.63	50		2007	133	111	40	108	173				
70	F							2708	207	129	42	391	249				
79	M			+CATH			39	2322	218	158	36	291	252	C5/O	Y		
61	M		5					2242	205	138	36	333	241				
66	M			1				2254	187	137	33	252	220	PRA40			
69	F	Y	4					2415	168	161	45	133	233				
58	M	Y					10	2146	158	98	43	302	201	C5			TRI
56	F	Y	5					2452	194	152	40	158	234				
57	F	Y	5					2157	150	129	41	103	191				
61	M	Y						2213	206	181	35	124	241			Y	W
52	F	Y						2694	229	202	61	137	290	C20			W
77	F			0	1.04	>75		2141	160	140	50	100	210			Y	W/TRI
75	M							2096	201	152	40	243	241				
76	M						40	2072	172	129	39	213	211	LES80	Y		
52	F	Y		0				2118	215	169	53	229	266				
75								2007	222	189	44	165	266				
67	F		3		0.7	50	NORMAL	2398	230	185	61	226	291				
75	F	Y	5	+CATH				2017	254	204	53	249	307	L10/O	Y		
54	M	Y						2021	121	99	32	110	153				
60								2188	255	N/C	69	599	325				
66								2271	211	169	38	210	249				
79								2020	148	129	54	96	202				
72	F							2151	183	156	53	140	236	C10			
65	F	Y						2428	328	N/C	46	1243	374				
77	M		3					2106	171	141	33	148	204				
62								2431	198	166	37	161	235				
89								2246	198	173	53	126	251				
89								2071	258	226	51	160	309				
61								2580	221	178	68	215	289				
61								2196	168	134	43	172	211				
92	F			391			39	2670	264	217	54	236	318	C10			
66	F							2020	209	189	54	100	263				
59								2259	209	189	44	102	253				
47								2087	215	174	57	203	272				
47								2075	199	161	40	190	239				
38								2296	219	181	12	168	231				
39								2063	159	N/C	41	437	200				
58	F		5	70				4073	281	221	48	301	329				
49								2044	194	N/C	42	446	236				
88	F							2007	128	115	57	84	185				

LDL-C: The Old Standard

As my mentor, Dr. Dayspring, would tell me, there is no test for LDL. It is a test for LDL-C or LDL cholesterol.

To complicate this, one has to ask if the LDL-C was calculated in a lipid panel or is it a direct measurement of LDL-C.

With a lipid panel, the patient must fast in order for the TG level to be low enough to allow the calculation of the LDL-C to be accurate.

A direct LDL-C can be done in a nonfasting patient. Apparently, it is not a good standardized test.

The great evidence-based trials have been done with LDL-C. The 4S trial and the HPS trial showed that lowering LDL-C lowers events and even mortality.

We don't have that evidence for HDL-C or triglycerides.

It is easy to understand why there is a great deal of resistance to changing the paradigm to following APOB or LDL-P, especially when to get the non-HDL cholesterol is almost as good as an APOB level.

I asked lipid expert Greg Brown in Miami why we didn't talk about the rhinoceros in the room—APOB. I said the JUPITER trial showed that LDL-C was in the normal range of less than 130 in patients with one risk factor. This allowed Crestor to be used head-to-head with a placebo. The post hoc data, however, showed that the APOB in these patients was 110 or in the 70th percentile. These were not low-risk patients. Clearly, APOB test will show us the real risk that patients have. Dr. Brown told me that APOB is not standardized. We were on our own if we used it. I did not have an opportunity for rebuttal. The LDL-C in the lipid panel is calculated, yet NCEP wants us to use that as the primary goal. The HDL-C of less than 40 is a major risk factor for heart disease, and yet it is not standardized and can be off 10% in local labs.

It is complicated already, and we need a new system. I have used LDL-P for the last year and have found that there were many patients who I thought I was treating to goal of LDL-C of less than 70, only to find they have discordance with the LDL-P and are not truly at goal. There are also the occasional patients who have very large LDL-Cs and their particle numbers are normal and they don't need further treatment.

LDL-P with NMR LipoScience lab allows me to treat to one number. I try to get the LDL-P less than 1,000 in high risk and less than 750 in very high risk. I don't worry what the LDL-C is. I don't spend time calculating the non-HDL cholesterol(Tubby Factor). Looking at one number is simpler than looking at LDL-C and non-HDL cholesterol(Tubby factor).

THE COMPLEX PUZZLE OF HDL

What is normal HDL-C? Less than 40 HDL-C is considered a major risk factor! The ADA advises raising HDL-C to more than 50.
Many physicians believe the higher the better.
My prediction is that the new NCEP guidelines NCEP will again not use HDL-C as a guideline goal. There is no drug that is presently indicated to raise HDL-C. The ARBITER 6 trial may bring more attention to this. Niacin raises the large HDL, and Trilipex raises the small HDL. Both seem to have better functionality, but they don't have that indication. Functionality is the key, and there is no commercial test to tell us if the HDL is functional or not. Torceptibid raised HDL-C, but the outcomes were worse. Milano syndrome has a low number of small HDLs which appear to extend the life of these patients.

Dr. Cromwell teaches that higher HDL-C is usually better. Thus, I try to give niacin to all my patients with a statin. If they already have a high HDL-C, I often use Zetia with a statin instead. With the ARBITER 6 trial, I will give niacin more preference; but in triple therapy, Zetia is still my third drug to get to LDL-P goal.

The very interesting point is that as HDL-C goes up to 45, the particle number usually increases. Above an HDL-C of 45, the particle number does not go up so much as the size of the HDL goes up. Some people that have a lot of very large HDL particles may actually give their cholesterol to the foam cells in the wall of the artery and make the disease worse.

Despite all the confusion, I still try to get my patients to an HDL-C of more than 50.

The great clinical pearl is that only 1,000 mg of niacin has to be given to get the greatest bang for the buck with raising HDL. Endur-acin is safe at 1,000 mg in terms of liver toxicity and glucose elevation. Endur-acin is $70 for a thousand pills if purchased online. I rarely have to stop Endur-acin because a patient complains of flushing.

For patients with the Tubby Factor, the good news is that strenuous exercise for one hour a day and weight loss can give tremendous elevations in HDL-C.

The Third Lipid You Need to Know About: Triglycerides

What is normal triglyceride level?
The physiological normal is 0-70 fasting.
"TG >136 with HDL-C <40 suggests the presence of the dangerous kind of VLDL (remnants) and most probably the most dangerous variety of LDL," as per William Castelli in *American Journal of Cardiology* (1992, 70:3h-9h) as reported in Dr. Daysprings' June 2009 blog.
I have no trouble getting my patients to TG of less than 100 with fish oil, so I do it.

Causes of Elevated Triglycerides:

> Excessive alcohol
> Cigarette smoking

High-carbohydrate diets (cruises)
Genetic disorders
Diabetes
Renal Disorders
Various drugs
Obesity
Lack of exercise

If you do not have any of the above, your TG should be from 10 to 70 or around 30. A TG of more than 200 is abnormal whether fasting or not.

NCEP states the following:

A normal fasting TG is less than 150.
TG 150-200 borderline CV risk
TG 200-500 high CV risk
TG > 500 very high risk with possible pancreatitis

If a patient has a TG more than 200, the NCEP secondary goal kicks in. Get the Tubby Factor (non-HDL cholesterol) less than 100 in very high-risk patients after getting the LDL-C to goal.

After getting LDL-P to goal, I try to get the TG to less than 100 with fish oil. Usually fish oil and Endur-acin get all my patients to TG less than 100.
After you take a cruise and gained 10 lb., go do a nonfasting TG level after eating pancakes. This is the Tubby Factor's stress test for TGs. It should be less than 200.

The low HDL-C with high TG have been undertreated for years because LDL-C is often normal at the same time. Look at my numbers back in 1993. I had a LDL-C less than 100 so I didn't take any medicine.

Now we know that I had elevated Tubby Factor because I had the Tubby syndrome. Subtract the HDL-C from the total cholesterol, and if it is greater than 80, a very high-risk patient needs treatment. Getting an LDL-P or APOB is even more accurate, but if you can't afford the advanced lipid testing, get your non-HDL cholesterol (Tubby Factor) to less than 80.

Non-HDL Cholesterol: The Tubby Factor

What is normal non-HDL cholesterol? The Tubby guidelines call for the Tubby Factor to be less than 80. The 2001/2003 NCEP guidelines state that for very high-risk patients the goal is less than 100 if TGs are more than 150. It is interesting that NCEP ignores non-HDL cholesterol (Tubby Factor) if the TGs are less than 150, and yet it is known that at high TG levels, the non-HDL cholesterol has discordance with APOB and LDL-P.

Non-HDL-C (Tubby Factor) is VLDL-C plus LDL-C. VLDLs are big fat balls and will not enter the arterial wall as readily.
VLDL-P is measured by NMR LipoProfile and included in the APOB immunoassay test. However, in patients with the Tubby syndrome, the VLDLs hang around longer and are larger. The particle is carrying more TG and cholesterol. This is why there is discordance between the amount of cholesterol and the amount of particles. The same number of particles will carry different amounts of cholesterol. Thus, the Tubby Factor measures the cholesterol amount while the NMR LipoProfile and the APOB immunoassay measure the number of particles. This is true for HDL-C and HDL-P as well. The particles are what carry the cholesterol into the artery wall and have been shown to be a more accurate predictor of disease.

I bet the next NCEP guidelines will make non-HDL cholesterol (Tubby Factor) the new primary goal, and they will lower it in very high-risk patients to 80 as per the new position paper AACC (American Association of Clinical Chemists 2009, *Clinical Chemistry*, 55:407-419).

Remember what Dr. Grundy wrote above; if the non-HDL cholesterol (Tubby Factor) is at goal, it does not matter what the LDL-C is. Thus, just disregard LDL-C and use the non-HDL cholesterol (the Tubby Factor). I advise this to be the goal even if the TG is not more than 150.

NMR LDL-P is a better test than Tubby Factor to predict heart disease. I use it all the time with my Medicare patients as Medicare pays for it. Most of my private insurance patients are not covered for NMR LipoProfile. I use the Tubby Factor for them, as it is simply a calculation based on the lipid panel.

The following is from the article "APOB versus Non-HDL-C: What to Do When They Disagree" by Allan Sniderman et al. from *Current Atherosclerosis Reports* (2009, 11:358-363).

"Discordance Between Non-HDL-C and APOB
The JUPITER trial.
LDL-C < 108 was at the 25th percentile
non-HDL-C 134 was at 30th percentile
APOB 109 was at the 60th percentile for men and 70th percentile for women.
"The discordance between the levels of LDL-C and non-HDL-C versus APOB is substantial by any measure."

"Diabetes and abdominal obesity, the disorders that promote discordance between APOB and non-HDL-C, are becoming more and more common, so APOB will become more and more useful."

"We must point out that APOB and non-HDL-C [*Tubby Factor*] measure different things.

  1- Each proatherogenic lipoprotein particle contains one particle of APOB.
  2- Therefore, measurement of APOB provides a precise estimate of the number of atherogenic particles whereas
  3- non-HDL-C equals [*Tubby Factor*] the sum of the mass of cholesterol and cholesterol ester within APOB particles."

Numbers and italics are mine.

VLDL-P

VLDL-C is triglycerides divided by 5.
Normal VLDL-C has been said to be 30 if TG of 150 is normal.
However if 100 is a normal TG level then normal VLDL-C is 20.

The VLDL-P are the big fat balls secreted from the liver. Their half-life is prolonged in diabetics and metabolic syndrome. They break down to remnants which are very atherogenic.

Chapter Sixteen

NIACIN (NICOTINIC ACID):
ONE DRUG THAT DOES IT ALL

Niacin

Endur-acin (sustained-release niacin) has been a great boon to my practice. When I first started treating lipids back in probably 1982, I could not get patients to take niacin or Niaspan because of the flushing. I could not get patients to take cholestyramine because of the grittiness and the constipation.

Presently, we have two great drugs. We have statins, and we have niacin in the form of Endur-acin. These are very well tolerated and very safe. Niacin does it all. It raises HDL-C; lowers LDL-C, TG, and APO (a); and makes LDL-P larger.

Endur-acin

An endocrinologist in Oklahoma was the first one to recommend Endur-acin to me. I read about Endur-acin in the Peter Kowalski book *8 Weeks to Lower Your Cholesterol.*

A cardiologist in Kansas City has used this in many of his patients and related his success with Endur-acin to me.

Endur-acin was studied in an article titled "Niacin Revisited: A Randomized Controlled Trial of Wax Matrix Sustain Released Niacin" (Kennan, J. et al. 1991, *Archives Internal Medicine*, 151:1414-1432).

Based on these endorsements, I cautiously began giving my patients Endur-acin. It rarely caused the side effect of flushing. This is critical for patient compliance. I now start at 500 mg BID with meals. Do not give 1,000 mg at one time. It is useful to break the tablet in half if you want to titrate slowly up or down. I usually stop at 1,000 mg because that's the safest for the liver and diabetes.

Do not give it to patients with gout, peptic ulcer disease, or intermittent atrial fibrillation.

It is often pointed out that HDL-C is not a NCEP guideline. However, the American Diabetic Association does advise to raise HDL-C in diabetics. Endur-acin is available on the Internet. Presently, you can buy a thousand tabs for $70.

For less that $90 a year, I can treat patients with simvastatin and Endur-acin. This is what gave birth to the Tubby theory:

We can prevent heart disease with simvastatin/Endur-acin in America for less than $90 a year if we find subclinical atherosclerosis early with CAC/ CIMT.

This is the key to combination therapy. Niacin has not been used much because of the flushing side effects. I have been able to put hundreds of patients on niacin in the form of Endur-acin. It is in a wax matrix and is sustained released. Slo-Niacin is similar and was used in very high doses in the HATS study, but I find Endur-acin has less flushing.

Important Points about Using Endur-acin

1. At 500 mg BID with meals, the HbA1c and the liver function tests are not significantly affected.
2. As per the *Seacoast trial,* you will get more LDL-C reduction with 1,000 mg of niacin than you will get with doubling your statin.
3. Only niacin and colestipol have the indication in combination in the PDR to regress plaque.
4. Don't take more than 750 mg of Endur-acin at one time.
5. Nonflush niacin is inactive on lipid profile.

Many Wonderful Studies

1. *The Coronary Drug Project* showed niacin 3g/d to *decrease total mortality* over a fifteen-year period by 11% and coronary mortality (Post ad hoc study 1986—1,119 people in the study—LDL-C was down 10% by year 1.)

2. CLAS I:
    One hundred sixty-two men had angiograms. The 16.2 % had regression of plaque with two drugs niacin/colestipol. The 2.4% in placebo group had regression. (P=0.002)

3. 1990 CLAS II:
    Nonprogression of plaque was 52% vs. 15% in placebo.
    Regression of plaque was 18% vs. 6% in placebo.
    (niacin 3-12 g a day given, 103 men had angiograms)
    Colestipol 30 g a day given

4. FATS: First major study to document regression 1990, angiogram study with about two hundred people in study
    Niacin/colestipol arm 36 men with LDL-C down 32% and HDL-C up 43% showed 39% regression of plaque.
    If LDL-C did not fall to less than 120, the niacin was increased to 1.5 g QID.

5. HATS:
    Slo-Niacin 1,000 mg BID (similar to Endur-acin) was used in this study. If HDL had not increased by 10 in twelve months, the patient was switched to crystalline niacin at 3 g a day. This was to avoid liver toxicity with the sustained-release niacin.
    Thirty-three people on niacin plus simvastatin in 10-20 mg range.
    LDL-C decreased 43%.
    HDL-C increased 26 %.
    Plaque regressed 0.4%/3%

The simvastatin/niacin plus *antioxidants* increased plaque 0.7%/7%. This is what stopped the vitamin E craze.

HATS was versus placebo.
The 149 patients with niacin/statin slowed progression over twelve months.
CIMT study with 149 patients
Statin + placebo 0.044-mm progression
Statin + niacin 0.0114-mm progression

ARBITER II trial: Extended-release nicotinic acid (Niaspan) 1,000 mg each was used. This was first clinical trial to show superiority of combination therapy *vs.* monotherapy.

This trial showed that when extended-release niacin was added to statin, combo therapy slowed the progression of carotid atherosclerosis over twelve months.

ARBITER III trial with CIMT on statin/niacin
With 149 patients in 2006 (study completed with 104 patients)
Twelve months with 125 patients showed 0.027-mm regression
Twenty-four months with fifty-seven patients showed 0.041-mm regression
Extended-release niacin 1,000 mg when added to statin, induced atherosclerosis regression measured by CIMT over twenty-four months
Limitations to this study include its open-label design and the inability to relate CIMT effects to clinical outcomes.

ARBITER VI
11-16-09
No surprises here. It's only about two hundred patients on niacin 2 g vs. Zetia. Both were given with statin. The starting LDL-C was in the eighties. Both arms had a subsequent drop to less than 70 LDL-C. HDL-C went up with niacin and went down with Zetia. However, this might mean nothing if both populations had the same HDL-P. The theory will be that the increase in HDL-C allowed more RCT (reverse cholesterol transport) out of the walls of the carotid artery. This is why niacin showed regression and Zetia did not. Niacin has always been my number 2 drug. Zetia will continue to be my number 3 drug to get patients to LDL-P goal. Ultimately, it is not about the surrogate marker of CIMT. I am not going to subject my patients to the side effects of 2 g of niacin. I prefer to give the 1 gram of Endur-acin and then add on Zetia. This no side-effect approach protects me from having skitist patients drop their medicine altogether when they get flushing from high-dose niacin.

Compell Study by McKenny J et al. (2007, *Atherosclerosis*, 192: 432-437)

Head-to-head study over twelve weeks

Four arms:	APOB	HDL-C	TG	Tubby Factor	
Atorvastatin/niacin ER 40mg/2,000mg	-43%	+22%	-47%	-55%	60 patients
Rosuvastatin/niacin ER 20mg/1,000	-42%	+24%	-40%	-49%	65 patients
Simvastatin/eszetimibe 40mg/10mg	-41%	+10%	-33%	-54%	72 patients
Rosuvastatin 40 mg	-39%	+7%	-25%	-43%	73 patients

For APOB, not much difference. *Notice that only 1,000mg of niacin is needed with Crestor 20 mg.*

For HDL-C and TG, niacin had a noticeable effect and again 1,000 mg gave the most bang for the buck.

In Dr. Dayspring's blog "Lipidaholics Anonymous Case 237: June 24, 2009," he writes:

> "Advicor and Simcor (simvastatin/Niaspan): neither has an FDA indication to reduce CV events due to lack of data."

> However PDR did note that simvastatin and colestipol in combination does have the indication for regression of plaque. What is a poor confused lipidologist like myself to do? With study and experience and lessons from other masters of lipidology I have found a *Tubby Treatment* that is inexpensive and finds disease early. Dr. Dayspring points out that the above studies are small and the doses of niacin are large in some of them. Some of the studies were done with Slo-Niacin which is a sustained release niacin similar to Endur-acin. In my studies when I learned that 1,000 mg of niacin will give me the best bang for the buck on HDL-C, I decided this is the drug for my Tubby syndrome (metabolic syndrome) patients. Over the years I slowly added the Endur-acin because I was concerned about the glucose going up. It has not been a problem so I now start patients off at the full dose of 500 mg twice a day with meals. The Seacoast trial had good lowering of LDL-C with simvastatin. This re-enforced my choice to give Endur-acin with statins.

Thanks to reading Lipidaholics, I learned there is *only one positive combination outcome trial*: Stockholm Ischemic Trial (Acta Med Scan 1988, 223:405-418). This was both a primary and secondary outcome study that was positive with Clofibrate and immediate-release niacin. This was a non-blinded study, and many of the patients were only on 1,500 mg of niacin.

No level 1 evidence for niacin, but *you gotta love this drug*. Endur-acin is a sustained-release niacin which at 1,000 mg has almost no flushing, no hepatic toxicity, and no increase in Hb A1c. Best of all, you can buy a thousand tabs of 500 mg for $70 on the Internet. Don't take it if you have gout.

Niacin:

1. Decreased total mortality by 11%
2. *FDA indication for plaque regression* with clofibrate
3. Primary and secondary outcome evidence with clofibrate
4. Raises HDL-C
5. Lowers triglycerides
6. Lowers LDL-C
7. Lowers lipoprotein (a)
8. Enlarges size of LDL-P

No other drug does all these things.

Zetia is a great drug for combo drug therapy. However, it cannot compare to the above data for niacin. Thus, I use niacin for combination therapy with statin before I use Zetia.

There is no level 1 outcome evidence for Zetia. However, the SEAS trial had a positive secondary end point to reduce ischemic events for Vytorin (simvastatin/Zetia). To me, that is very significant. Zetia also had good CIMT results in the SANDS trial. This is a very good drug to get to LDL-P goal. We have to wait until 2012 for the Improve-it trial for level 1 evidence.

In my NLA-SAP booklet (volume 3, page14), it states the following:

> Niacin 1,000 mg/d increases HDL by 20% with more increase in the large HDL vs. the small HDL.

> Fenofibrate increases small-size HDL and decreases large size HDL.

> Actos increases HDL by 14%.

Chapter Seventeen

ZETIA: THE MUCH MALIGNED DRUG

Despite several negative trials, this is still a good drug. It has a positive secondary outcome in the SEAS trial, and it did well with CIMT in the SANDS trial but recently it lost to niacin in a head-to-head trial, Arbiter 6. Look closely at the results of Arbiter 6. There was no progression of atheroma with Zetia and a little insignificant regression. The media seems to have missed this point.

I still believe it is safer to use a moderate dose of a statin and then add on a second drug rather than go to maximum monotherapy with the statin. In my experience, taking a patient to maximum statin dose increases the risk of myalgias, which may turn a patient away from statins for a long time. In my practice, I will start off with low-dose statin in order to avoid myalgias. I also worry that my elderly patients might continue the statins despite becoming ill and thus risk rhabdomyolysis. I prefer to use Endur-acin as the second drug at 500 mg BID. I then will add the third drug Zetia to get to LDL-P goal of less than 750. I find patients tolerate these three drugs quite well.

If a patient has a HDL-C of more than 50 after starting the moderate dose of statin, I will go to Zetia directly. Subsequent to Arbiter 6 trial, I might pay more attention to the HDL-P and go to Endur-acin if the HDL-P is less than 30 with a HDL-C of more than 50.

In recent months, I have found several patients have a creeping elevation of LDL-P on statin monotherapy. I presume these are patients that compensate the decreased production of LDL-P in the liver by absorbing more cholesterol from the bile in the gut. It makes sense to thus block that absorption with Zetia.

There is the occasional patient who does not respond well to statin monotherapy. These are probably hyperabsorbers of cholesterol. I would advise backing down to minimal statin dose and adding Zetia to these patients.
The Improve-it trial will hopefully give us a positive primary outcome with Zetia. I am not going to fail reaching LDL-P goal in the meantime by avoiding Zetia.

I imagine some physicians will give maximum statin and then increase niacin until they reach LDL-P goal. I find that fraught with patient noncompliance.

Chapter Eighteen

STATINS: THE KING OF DRUGS

In memory of Tim Russert, I started making YouTube videos to better inform the public about preventing heart attack and stroke. In 2008, I was advancing my knowledge of lipidology when Mr. Russert died, and not much was made of how he was treated and the details of his case. I felt more could be said, and this was a golden opportunity to teach the public about what is available and what can be done. Instead, I heard that cases like this are inevitable—well, there are 100,000 cases of sudden death outside of the hospital every year, and my goal is with primary prevention to prevent it. Some people have asked why my YouTube approach is so informal. Well, in memory of Tim Russert, when he used a little board that said Florida, Florida, Florida, I also want to deliver a similar easy message. It's information, not style. It is STATINS, STATINS, STATINS!

This is the story folks, it's statins, statins, statins. I know there are reluctant patients out there, and it's the reluctant patients that make doctors relax and not push for aggressive therapy. For the reluctant patient, I can simply point out that aspirin is available over the counter, and it is really the best treatment to prevent sudden death. However, one in fifty thousand people bleed from this. This is a dangerous drug in comparison to statins. Statins—their record shows one in one million people for cases of rhabdomyolisis.

Some patients like to use red yeast rice instead of Lipitor because it is natural and cheaper. This is a big mistake as evidenced by the following example of the blood thinner Coumadin or warfarin. These drugs are used in rat poison, so for those people who like to take things that are off-label (not reviewed by the FDA), they might go into the hardware store and say, "Oh, just give me some rat poison since it's the same thing." Well, how much do you take? Patients may not know whether to take one or two tablespoons of rat poison, but they seem to think they know the dose for red yeast rice. You have to understand that the FDA does not test natural products. There is no way to know (other than testimonials from friends) about how much to take or what you are doing to yourself. That is how the Brooklyn Bridge has been sold many times to out-of-towners. With that said, I think we must have enormous respect for all drugs. There is *no* such thing as a perfectly safe drug, and patients have to realize that when they take a drug there is no total guarantee.

People don't realize that Advil has a black box warning for stroke and heart attack ever since the Vioxx debacle.

Baychol was a problem; of course it was used in high dose in combination with Gemfibrozil. This combination turned out to be deadly.

Avoid Zocor at 80 mg, it's probably also an unsafe dose.

Clofibrate was found to be toxic and had to be taken off the market.

Triparanol was a scandal. I'll let you look that up with Google.

The Case for Regular Visits

Despite the dark history of the examples above, I still say treat aggressively. Find disease and get their LDL particle number at least under 1,000 if not under 750 and monitor at least three times a year. Patients often give us a hard time and want to come in just once a year. I think this is a very big mistake. I see a great deal of hypothyroidism, which can lead to rhabdomyolisis. As patients get older, their renal function decreases, which can be a very big problem for Zocor or simvastatin. If they have muscle pain, I get the CPK. This is mostly to convince the patient that they are *not* having rhabdomyolisis and that they simply need to cut back on the statin and try to work with it. Often I find that the vitamin D level is low, and I get this level before I start statins to avoid the whole problem of muscle pain.

Treating aggressively is not really what the guidelines are about. The guidelines are actually the minimum, the benchmark from which physicians should work. They give a great deal of leeway for the physician to use his judgment. My judgment is that if you have artery disease, as demonstrated in previous chapters, then you need to prevent sudden death and to stabilize that plaque, no matter how small that plaque is. I would also like to see regression of plaque.

What to Do If You Can't Take Statins

The most common referral from primary care physicians to me in my lipid clinic is to treat their patients who state they cannot take statins.

Here is what I do.

I order a vitamin D level, CPK level, SED rate and CRPhs and NMR LipoProfile, glucose, creat, BUN, and AST, if they have not been done recently.

I find out which statins they tried and what exact symptoms they had on the statin and whether they had those symptoms before or after the statins.

Did they try very low dose statin such as Crestor 5 mg once a week?

Did they have a vitamin D level done? If I find the level is low, I will give vitamin D 50,000 IU once a week for eight weeks before I start statins again. I will often check the vitamin d level again as well. While they are off statins, I will start patient on fish oil and Endur-acin or Zetia.

Once the vitamin D level is done, I will try Crestor 5 mg or Lipitor 10 mg once a week.

At this point, I hope the patient is on Crestor 5 mg once a week and Endur-acin 500 mg BID with meals. After two months, I check the NMR LipoProfile.

If no pain, I go to Crestor 5 mg Monday, Wednesday, Friday with Endur-acin.

After two months, I check the NMR LipoProfile and may have to add Zetia at this point.

In two months after taking Crestor 5 mg Monday, Wednesday, and Friday and Endur-acin BID and Zetia QD, I check their level again.

If triglycerides are high, I switch to high-dose Lovaza and later add Trilipex if needed.

If LDL-P is still high and TGs are okay, I will add Welchol two tabs BID with meals.

Two months later, if LDL-P is still high, I can increase the Welchol or switch patient to Niaspan and increase the niacin to 2,000 mg a day.

If the patient can't take Crestor once a week, I try Lipitor once a week. If they can't take that, I try Leschol XL 80 once a day. If that fails, I try pravastatin low dose once a day.

I believe we can get the patient close to goal with a low dose of some type of statin if we are persistent and follow the CPKs at the time we stop the statin due to muscle pain.

Chapter Nineteen

FISH OIL TO FIGHT INFLAMMATION

This is a no-brainer. Everyone should take fish oil. The JELIS trial showed that the Japanese benefitted from taking DHA pills, and they already had a high fish intake.

Fish oil plus statins decrease the CRPhs by more than 70%. CRPhs measures inflammation. It is not clear to me that Tim Russert was on fish oil. His triglyceride level was very high. He would have benefitted with four tablets of Lovaza, and if that didn't get his TGs down, he could have gone up to six tablets a day.

Lovaza is the only FDA-approved fish oil. Everything else you take over the counter is guesswork in terms of what you are actually ingesting. The biggest side effect of taking OTC fish oil is calories. You usually end up with a lot of fish oil that is not the essential EPA/DHA.

Look at the back of your fish-oil bottle. Add up the DHA and the EPA. It should be at least 850 mg. This is what one tablet of Lovaza contains. The OTC pills usually require at least two tablets to reach the required 850 mg. That calculates out to eight tabs a day to get to the minimum dose to lower triglycerides.

The GISSI trial prevented sudden death with only 850 mg of DHA/EPA. The only down side is the fish burp. It is just a nutritional supplement.
I don't worry about the equivocal studies in patients with implanted defibrillators. There are positive and negative studies in small numbers of patients.

I have had cardiologists stop the fish oil tabs because of pill burden. I can't agree with that. We learned with HIV patients with AIDS that taking ten pills a day is often required and patients manage the pill burden when they want to do better. Many of the patients who complain of pill burden are taking handfuls of vitamins and gingkos and saw palmetto and garlic and cinnamon. Fish oil has prevented sudden death. That is not the pill to stop. Stop the Advil and Aleve. Those pills have black box warnings. We have many young patients with metabolic syndrome(Tubby syndrome). Yes, they should lose weight and exercise, but until they do that, they will need to take several pills a day. Diabetics have to take a minimum of four to ten pills when they first walk in the door. These pills are evidence based and very safe. The most dangerous pill is always the baby aspirin they need to take.

Chapter Twenty

COMBINATION THERAPY

A high dose of statins is safe especially with Lipitor as shown in the TNT trial. For people who have more money, my preference is Crestor. For people who are older with some questionable renal insufficiency, my preference is Lipitor. Since you only get a 6% decrease by increasing your statin from moderate to the highest dose, I think it is better to just add a 1,000 mg of niacin, which will decrease the LDL-C by 12%. So here you get double the effect with much less risk. Simvastatin 80 mg, I think, is high risk in terms of developing rhabdomyolisis.

I think that Endur-acin is a great drug, and I think there is evidence that shows that it is the best drug for regression of plaque. I think it is also shown you can also get regression of plaque if you can get the LDL-C under 76 by IVUS studies.

I think that for diabetics, Welchol is a good second or third drug as it lowers hemoglobin A1c. I love Zetia because I think it will give you a great punch at lowering your particle number. Welchol, Zetia, even Trilipix (which is a great drug for diabetics)—all of those are very expensive, and there are no outcome studies with those three drugs. Now there are outcome studies with gemfibrozil which is very similar to Trilipix, and there are outcome studies for cholestyramine which is very similar to Welchol. But there are no real true outcomes studies for Zetia yet.

Important safety tip—I would not go over 1,500 mg of Enduracin nor Slo-Niacin. There is one article for Endur-acin and that is the highest dose they used. The package insert for Endur-acin says do not use more than 750 mg per dose, so I give this twice a day at 500 mg with meals.

I think you should monitor LFT or AST three times a year along with the glucose. Even though the glucose may fluctuate up a little bit, I think you will see that the hemoglobin A1C does not change. I would avoid niacin in uncontrolled diabetes, as well as gout, peptic ulcer disease, or atrial fibrillation.

Simvastatin, you have to love this drug because it is generic. However, I am really concerned for the patient with some renal insufficiency or someone who gets very sick. If the patient gets very sick on you, please stop the statin. Rhabdomyolisis is rare at one in a million. We don't want to see any cases in our practice, and if you are going to get a problem with rhabdomyolisis, it is going to be on simvastatin 80 mg in patient who gets sick. Their renal function decreases, or they take other drugs which cause the level to go up, and then they may get rhabdomyolisis. I often find that muscle pain is associated with the vitamin D level, so I always get vitamin D levels, and if the level is under 32, then give the patient 50,000 IU once a week for eight weeks and then 2,000 IU a day. I probably check the vitamin D after that in the wintertime.
Avoid the high-dose 80 mg simvastatin. Watch for drug interaction, especially with erythromycin and verapamil.

I have no financial interest in Endur-acin. I speak for many companies. I only promote Endur-acin and simvastatin to offer an inexpensive treatment. I think they are very safe drugs, but I think many of these drugs are very safe. Actually, the combination of Simvastatin with Niaspan in Simcor might be a drug for Medicaid patients. In my Topeka, Medicaid will pay for it, and the patient will then be able to get the two drugs while they could not afford the $16 for one hundred tablets of over-the-counter Endur-acin which Medicaid would not pay for.
I think combination therapy is the way to go for safety and for efficacy.

NMR LipoProfile Case Studies

These are NMR LipoScience LipoProfiles. These are what I obtain for patients to see what their LDL particle number is. The reason I do this will be demonstrated in the next two cases. I often find discordance between the LDL-C number and the LDL particle number.

Case 1

In this first case, a sixty-nine-year-old female diabetic on Crestor 10 mg and Zetia 10 mg with a hemoglobin A1C of 6.6. She has rheumatoid arthritis which is a risk factor for heart disease. The best way to treat this patient to prevent heart disease is to put the patient on methotrexate. For some reason, this patient is not on methotrexate right now. Rheumatoid arthritis is an inflammatory disease, and this inflammation affects the coronary arteries.

However, in order to do what we can do in the lipid clinic, we will check her LDL particle number and compare it to her LDL-C. Her particle number is 1,015, which is higher than what you would think with the LDL-C calculated of 65 and the LDL-C direct of 56. The LDL-C calculated is not very accurate. The LDL direct may be more accurate, but there are many more artherogenic particles as demonstrated by the LDL particle number of 1,015. The patient's triglyceride level is pretty good. Her HDL-C is also fairly good at 58. Thus, this is a patient who is diabetic, and we don't really want to give her Welchol because her hemoglobin A1C is already 6.5. The Welchol would lower her hemoglobin A1C by 0.5, and we don't really want to give her Tricor because her triglycerides are okay. Niacin is a possibility, but her HDL-C is really pretty good and doesn't seem to be the best way to go. She is already on Zetia, so I think for this lady the best way to treat her is to increase her Crestor to 20 mg a day. This will decrease her LDL particle number hopefully to below 750. She is high risk because she is diabetic.

Case 2

Here is another lady exhibiting discordance. She is an eighty-two-year-old female on simvastatin. She is a diabetic, and her hemoglobin A1C is not very well controlled at 8.5 Her nuclear stress test was a poor study, but normal in 2002. Now this might be a good lady for Welchol because it would lower her hemoglobin A1C by at least 0.5 However, this lady has a slightly elevated triglyceride level at 169. Thus, this might be a good lady to give Tricor to because it will also raise her low HDL-C from 41 to hopefully above 50.

As you can see, this lady does have discordance, as her particle number is 1,186 and her LDL-C calculated is 51. Normally, no one would ever think of adding on medications to this lady because her LDL-C is 51; however, once we get the LDL particle number, we discover that she still has a lot of artherogenic particles.

There is discordance between the LDL particle number and the LDL-C. We need to be more aggressive. Thus, this lady is someone whom we might add Welchol. However, I think that Trilipex might be best because of the HDL-C and because Trilipex has such good evidence for helping microvascular disease.

Case 3

This patient is a sixty-seven-year-old male who has metabolic syndrome(Tubby syndrome) and a Framingham risk of 25%. The Framingham risk puts him at high risk, and the metabolic syndrome in addition to that puts him at very high risk.

He's on simvastatin 40 mg each night, Endur-acin which is niacin 500 mg twice a day, fish oil 2,000 mg a day. He had a negative treadmill and, as we know, could still have quite a bit of disease and the plaque can rupture. His LDL particle number, interestingly enough, is 1,032, but because he is a very high-risk patient, I think we should definitely get his particle number below 750.
This is a case where the LDL-C calculated is 69, and again we see discordance here. Most people would have stopped with this LDL of 69 and felt comfortable. Indeed, Tim Russert had an LDL-C of 68. We see that in this very high-risk patient we are not at goal on the LDL particle number, and we need to give him something more.

He's already on simvastatin. I suggested that we could increase the simvastatin to 80 mg and make sure he takes it at night. But I would only suggest that if this is a patient who can't afford lipitor or crestor or goes to the VA and that's all they will give him. I would prefer to switch him to Crestor 20 mg, but the patient wants to go on generic. I have a lot of concerns about 80 mg of simvastatin. I think the risk for toxicity is great.

Case 4

A seventy-three-year-old male who had a positive nuclear stress test and a slightly low ejection fraction of 36%. He's on simvastatin 40 mg a day. Again, the generic is nice, and in our neighborhood, it is $10 for three months at Walmart. His LDL particle number actually looks pretty good at 977. Now this is very important because with an LDL-C of 90 we would have wanted to treat him further. Going from 40 mg to 80 mg would have dropped him 6% on the simvastatin. However, we see that he is almost at goal here, where he's 977 (under 1,000). Thus, we are saving the patient the excess statin by getting the LDL particle number. His HDL-C is a little low at 44, so I would probably feel better to put this patient on Endur-acin 500 twice a day to get his particle number down. This would also raise his HDL-C.

Chapter Twenty-One

MAY YOU LIVE AS OLD AS MOSES

Age	sex	DM	Met Syn	CAC	CIMT	cimt%	Carotid Stenosis	LDLp	NON-HDL	LDLc	HDL	TG	Total CHOL	Statin	Enduracin	Zetia	Wel/Tri
98								1436	124	112	43	60	167				
98								1331	121	103	35	89	156				
97								1090	135	111	48	119	183				
95								939	84	67	77	87	161				
95								761	56	50	60	31	116				
95	M			104			39	660	56	50	43	31	99	L10	Y		
95	M							623	55	48	53	33	108				
94								1214	138	120	69	91	207				
94								835	121	101	60	102	181				
94								832	73	56	46	84	119				
94	M							819	77	67	37	48	114				
94								660	63	47	62	80	125				
93	F						39	1235	71	59	56	62	127	L40	Y	Y	
93	F		5				+	1213	108	93	83	77	191	C10		Y	
93	F							1178	79	63	60	78	139				
93	F					9		1103	96	74	33	110	129	S20	Y		
93								1011	91	72	60	93	151				
93	F							726	49	36	57	65	106				
93							39	648	83	64	82	97	165				
93								558	100	75	72	126	172				
92	F			391			39	2870	264	217	54	236	318				
92	F						74	1162	130	113	52	86	182	S20			
92	F		5					1048	86	72	63	68	149				
92	F			+CATH				918	103	79	67	118	170	S20			
92	F		5					886	72	60	78	62	150				
92	F		5					804	98	77	74	103	172				
92	F			374			9	623	66	52	58	71	124	C5/O	Y		
92	F							600	68	53	60	77	128				
92								528	103	84	70	95	173				
92	F							527	57	51	49	30	106				
91	M							1106	115	101	43	71	158				
91	F		5					1096	106	94	66	61	172				
91	M			0				1095	104	88	37	80	141	L10	Y		
91	F			3563			49	1006	94	59	52	175	146	C5/WK			
91	F							999	95	83	63	59	158				
91								968	75	60	40	74	115				
91	F							902	76	45	51	154	127				
91	M							887	93	78	41	73	134				
91	M							635	62	42	47	101	109	L20			
91	F							506	70	60	54	48	124				
90	M							1955	192	129	39	316	231				
90	F							1810	200	184	63	79	263				
90	F							1236	100	91	72	45	172				
90	M							1228	105	85	42	99	147				
90								1194	110	78	45	162	155				
90	F							1172	129	116	71	64	200				
90								1111	90	72	47	88	137				
90	F						39	1046	88	80	75	41	163	C5			
90								1015	96	77	53	96	149				
90	F			PVD				1004	113	99	76	70	189	L20			
90								973	129	105	62	122	191				
90	M	Y						863	69	28	32	207	101				
90	F							848	125	112	70	67	195				
90	F						59	780	97	73	66	122	163	C5			
90	M	Y						756	62	35	31	137	93				
90	M	Y		+CATH			80	697	66	19	37	234	103	S20	Y	Y	
89								2246	198	173	53	126	251				
89								2071	258	226	51	160	309				
89								1917	271	250	59	103	330				
89								1604	131	116	34	77	165				
89	M							1092	96	75	53	106	149				
89	F						39	947	88	78	67	51	155	C10			
89	M						39	820	103	80	60	116	163	C10			
89	F							807	99	87	67	61	166				
89	M							779	95	72	52	117	147				
89	F			+			39	749	78	63	74	75	152	L40	Y		
89	F							737	93	58	73	174	166				

Age	sex	DM	Met Syn	CAC	CIMT	cimt%	Carotid Stenosis	LDLp	NON-HDL	LDLc	HDL	TG	Total CHOL	Statin	Enduracin	Zetia	Wel/Tri
89	F							732	81	59	79	109	160				
89	F							625	75	49	71	129	146				
89								520	72	51	83	105	155				
88	F							2007	128	115	57	64	185				
88	F							1707	136	116	47	101	183				
88	M							1428	123	75	31	241	154				
88	F			200			39	1204	99	90	66	43	165	C20	Y		
88	F			1266				1189	75	65	51	48	126	P10			W
88	F							1182	107	91	69	78	176				
88	F							1093	75	66	70	45	145				
88	F						39	856	67	57	57	52	124	L20		Y	
88	F							849	78	60	56	92	134				
88	F			+ CATH			49	830	55	48	63	34	118	S10	Y		
88	F							819	103	91	71	58	174				
88					+		positive	788	48	42	40	31	88				
88	F							754	90	56	69	170	159				
88	F				+		39	694	92	21	44	354	136	S40	Y		
88	F			841			49	690	69	52	58	83	127	C20			
88	M							607	76	52	37	121	113				
88	F			410			39	607	78	61	97	83	175				
88								605	84	53	70	154	154				
88	M				+		39	591	53	36	40	87	93	S20	Y		
88	F							577	88	67	65	104	153				
87								1813	168	152	59	78	227				
87	F							1578	146	130	49	80	195				
87								1368	62	56	27	29	89				
87	F							1362	105	47	38	289	143				
87	F							1358	116	98	49	91	165				
87	F						39	1317	124	110	59	71	183	C5	Y		
87	F							1222	120	110	71	49	191				
87	M							1162	120	107	56	66	176				
87	M							1134	141	132	71	46	212				
87	F	3		656			9	1129	146	132	75	68	221	-			
87	F							1080	128	118	62	49	190				
87	F						39	1045	79	66	59	63	138	L20			
87	F							1008	90	79	71	53	161				
87	M						39	987	96	89	59	35	155				W
87	F							979	87	74	68	64	155				
87	F							959	73	62	56	53	129				
87	F							947	100	39	37	307	137				
87	F							925	95	82	57	67	152				
87	F							922	83	68	54	74	137				
87	F	3						861	128	114	80	72	208	S20			
87	M							739	59	53	49	31	108				
87								712	76	66	35	50	111				
87	F			+CATH				698	92	66	78	130	170	L40			
87	F							674	48	33	74	76	122				
87								672	66	56	38	51	104				
87	F							625	80	57	94	113	174				
87								584	63	57	56	32	119				
87								566	52	38	60	68	112				
87	M							561	92	59	43	165	135				
87								541	68	57	44	57	112				
87	M							519	55	47	53	38	108				
87	M						39	456	52	44	57	40	109	S40	Y		
87	F								99	69	41	69	140				
86	F						9	1307	106	90	52	80	158				
86	F							1011	87	76	57	57	144				
86	F	Y		+			70	968	100	87	50	65	150				
86	M							963	83	71	56	59	139				
86	F						9	926	83	74	68	44	151	L80			
86	M						40	915	76	61	57	76	133	S40		Y	
86	F						9	915	78	69	67	43	145				
86								892	128	111	56	83	184				
86	F							889	71	59	79	61	150				
86	M							877	63	57	49	32	112				
86	F	Y			+		70	838	97	78	56	93	153				

Recently there was a post hoc analysis of the JUPITER trial. It showed that you had to treat nineteen low-risk elderly before one patient received benefit from the highest dose of Crestor.

It makes sense, as older people are more at risk of a cardiac event. Statin trials show that the best results occur in people at highest risk. I refer to the TNT trial which had 98% risk reduction in the oldest patients with the highest risk.

Yet I am often derided by medical nihilists for treating the very elderly. One of our cardiovascular surgeons told me that he does thirty heart valve repairs a year in Topeka. I thought that was a lot. He said as the population gets older, the valves wear out; and as the elderly come to him in overall better health, they usually do well with valve replacement in their eighties. If we are not going to ration heart valve replacements in the elderly, I don't think $90 a year for simvastatin and Endur-acin is going to bust the bank. It certainly has been shown to help them.
The great physician Osler said pneumonia was the old man's friend as it gave him an easy death. When Osler became elderly, he called it the old man's enemy.

The number needed to treat(NNT) in patients aged at least seventy years treated with Crestor 40 for five years to prevent one primary composite end point (nonfatal MI or stroke), hospitalization for unstable angina or arterial revascularization was 19. The *Internal Medicine News* quotes Dr. Glynn of Brigham and Women's Hospital in Boston as saying, "JUPITER provides convincing evidence for the benefit of statin therapy in older individuals in the context of primary prevention . . . . on the absolute scale (as opposed to RRR or reduced relative risk), which is critical for treatment decisions, the treatment benefits were larger in older individuals." This was reported in volume 42, number 16 of the *Internal Medicine News* on September 15, 2009. This news from JUPITER should replace the Prosper trial data which did not show benefit of statin in the elderly for primary prevention.

In the SAGE trial (the Study Assessing Goals in the Elderly), a significant total mortality benefit was observed in elderly subjects with CHD who received atorvastatin 80 mg compared to pravastatin 40 mg.

In the five-year HPS trial, there were 5,806 persons aged 70 to 80 that had an absolute benefit greater in those aged older than seventy years old.

In the book *Clinical Challenges in Lipid Disorders* by Peter Toth and Dominic Sica, treating the elderly is well covered in their last chapter written by J. G. Robinson, MD, from the University of Iowa.

Chapter Twenty-Two

EXERCISE

100% commitment
100% responsibility

I read these words in Jack Canfield's book *The Success Principles*, and it helped me realize that I had to make a commitment to get up earlier and eat a four-hundred-calorie breakfast at 6:00 am. Then I had to go down to the YMCA and work out for an hour. I have done this faithfully since March 17, 2006, when I signed a contract with myself to lose 50 lb. I found the *3-Hour Diet* by Jorge Cruise, and I have continued to eat every three hours ever since. I lost 80 lbs. by June 2007 in time for my wedding. I have since gained back 45 lb. as of today, October 24, 2009. I had hit the plateau in June 2007. I couldn't lose any more weight. I decided to gain some weight back and regain much of the muscle mass I had lost. I decided the way to fight the plateau was to have the muscle to burn off the fat. Subsequently at the comprehensive cardiometabolic risk reduction program that I took at the Midwest NLA meeting in Cincinnati in September 2009, I was astonished by the fact that Dr. Louis Aronne taught. He said that *with 10% body weight loss, there is a 42% decrease in energy expenditure by muscles*.

The Amish study showed that the people with Tubby syndrome maintained weight loss by exercising off 900 calories a day.

The key point is that exercise is very important, but not as important as portion control and keeping calories below two thousand a day.

These are hard facts, but once we know the facts, we know what we need to do. We need a new way of thinking about what normal eating and normal exercise is.

I used to think a one-mile walk a day was pretty good. I usually lifted weight three times a week when I was into my exercise routine.

I now realize that I probably need to exercise an hour after each major meal. I have done that after breakfast at the YMCA, and after lunch, I usually walk for one hour. I still was able to eat more than I could burn especially since I had plateaued, and the exercise was not burning as many calories as I thought they should.

I still exercise twice a day and try to do more core-strength exercises. I eat more protein especially as my in-between-meal-two-hundred-calorie snack. Usually an Atkins protein bar or an Atkins vanilla protein shake.

I hope to get down to at least 220 lbs., which is where the original contract goal was.

I tell my story here to emphasize how difficult exercise and diet are, and if you have failed before, don't despair. Keep trying. It is over the long term that matters, and even an eight-minute walk a day makes a difference.

Start slow with eight-minute walks. In the morning when you wake up, pull your knees to your chest and stretch easily for twenty seconds.

From this starting point, slowly increase your activity.
If you do not do one session of exercise first thing in the morning, you will probably fail.
After a period of time, you will always find excuses to not exercise later in the day. If you make the morning exercise period a non-negotiable item in your schedule, you are much more likely to take the next step and eat a better diet.

As with eating, do an exercise you enjoy. Don't torture yourself with exercise that hurts or you find unbearable. Just move.

Chapter Twenty-Three

DIET

Diet is the deal breaker in the Tubby syndrome.

I lost 80 lb. two years ago and have gained back 45 lb. from July 1, 2007, till today October 20, 2009. I exercise two hours a day. I eat every three hours. I am not discouraged. I have the habit of eating every three hours, and I have the habit of exercising right after breakfast and walking an hour at lunch. I know that I will slowly lose the weight. I am hoping that this time I will not lose my muscle mass and thus I will prevent the plateau that occurs with the resultant turnoff of the metabolism.

My esteemed and beloved mentor, Dr. Thomas Dayspring, writes in October 2009 Lipidholics blog, "Lots of proven diets: Mediterranean, South Beach, Dash-with serious exercise *should* all be of benefit" (italics mine).

These diets are beautiful, the NCEP guidelines are beautiful. The amount of thought and evidence-based science that has gone into them is awesome.

The problem is they don't work. There are 100,000 sudden deaths in America and the Tubby syndrome (metabolic syndrome) in the population is an epidemic.

I am in clinical practice. I need something that works. Making a guideline to LDL-P of less than 1,000 doesn't work. Patients and doctors will look at an LDL-P of 1,100 and say that close enough for government work. That may be a good month when they took their medicine because they knew they were going to see the doctor. They miss the next appointment in four months because the last test was good enough, and they don't want to pay the $25 deductible for the office visit. Or it is a nice day out or it is a bad day out. None of this is in the guidelines. When the Prove-it trial says LDL-C goal was 70 and they had good outcomes, doctors forget half of those people were with LDL-C of with less than 70. When the JUPITER trial shows good outcomes with LDL-C of 55, doctors forget many of those patients went as low as LDL-C of 35. This is why I try to get my patients to less than 750 LDL-P to regress plaque. We may not get there with two drugs, but if we get to LDL-P of 800 with two drugs, I am satisfied. I will go to three or more drugs to get there in those patients who have had stents or bypasses.

Back to diet. As I tried to state a reasonable approach to the Tubby guideline of LDL-P of less than 750, there needs to be a reasonable approach to weight. Normal BMI is not reasonable for the Tubby population. Neither is ideal body weight or what you weighed when you were in high school. I don't even think a waist of forty inches for men or thirty-five inches for women may be reasonable in many cases. Don't set yourself or your patients up for failure.

Of course people will lose tremendous weight. They almost always gain it back. The fat cells don't go away. They are just waiting for a metabolic slow-plateau patient to go above 2,000 calories as I did. The weight comes back on.

Do what I did.

Eat every three hours.

Exercise after breakfast and after lunch.

Eat food you like but learn portion control.

If you can't use the King Calorie Book to weigh your food and write down everything you eat, then follow my Tubby Factor diet that I have below. You may not use it all the time, but try it for a day at a time to learn portion control. It is not tofu and it is not gourmet but it is right there in the freezer.

If you have salt-sensitive hypertension or congestive heart failure, I would not follow these prepared food diets.

I think the Tubby Factor diet is a good teaching tool. The boxes list all the ingredients. Learn to read the labels. If you are in a hurry, these are good to have in your freezer. This is for the people who say they don't have the time. This is for people who don't have the discipline to be mindful of everything they eat. They have more than the 7% saturated fat, but if you lose weight and are on statin, I don't think you need to worry about the extra saturated fat. People lose weight on the Atkins diet and have a lipid neutral effect on their lipid panels. The Mediterranean diet typically has 10-20 g of saturated fat. Some of the saturated fat in the Tubby syndrome diet is stearic acid which is lipid neutral. There is no trans-fatty acid in this diet. The Mediterranean diet has 20-30 g of fiber a day. Guidelines shoot for less than 2.4 g of sodium a day or 6 g/d sodium chloride intake.

Tubby Diet

1850 calorie diet for people > 250 pounds: (7% of diet is 130 calories or 14.4 g of saturated fat)

6AM	Aunt Jamina Ham and Egg Scramble	260 calories	13 g fat (3.5 saturated)	920 mg sodium	
	Weight Watchers Yogurt	100 calories	0.5 g fat (0 fat)	110 mg Na	6 g protein
	Fusion light 6 oz	38 calories			
9 AM	Snickers Marathon Protein Bar	290 calories	10g fat (5.0 sat fat)	190 na	20g protein
Noon	Banquet Spaghetti and Meatballs	400 calories	17 g fat (7.0 sat fat)	940 mg na	
3pm	Healthy Choice Chicken Artichoke Panini	300 calories	4 g fat (1.5 g sat fat)	600 mg na	
6 PM	Stouffer's Meatloaf	340 calories	19 g fat (8 g sat fat)	780 mg na	
	Large salad with Briannas Santa Fe Blend dressing				
	4 table spoons of salad dressing	50 calories			
9 PM	Lindt Excellenc 85% Cocoa one square	50 calories	5 g fat (4 g saturated fat) (stearic fatty acid has neutral		
				effect on lipids)	
	Total cal 1850 total	sat fat 25 g sat fat		4,300 mg Na	

1650 calorie diet for people > 200 pounds (7% of diet is 116 calories or 13 g of saturated fat)

6 AM	Jimmy Dean Muffin Sandwich Bacon,				
	Egg, Cheese	230 calories	9 g fat (3.5 g sat fat)	670 mg Na	
	Kraft Bagel-fuls whole grain				
	with cream cheese	180 calories	6 g fat (3.5 g sat fat)	200 mg Na	
9 AM	Adkins Advantage Chocolate				
	Chip Granola Bar	200 calories	8g fat (4 g sat fat)	190 mg Na	17 g protein
Noon	Marie Callenders Beef and Broccoli	400 calories	14 g fat (4.5 g sat fat)	1,200 mg Na	
			(beef has stearic fatty acid)		
3 PM	Crown Prince Kipper Snacks	190 calories	13 g fat (2g sat fat)	390 mg Na	19 g protein
6 PM	Banquet Chicken and Broccoli Pot Pie	350 calories	20g fat (9 g sat fat)	800 mg Na	
	Large salad with	45 calories			
	Neuman's Own Light Balsamic Vinaigrette				
	2 tablespoons				

9 PM	Apple	70 calories		
	Total approx	1650 calories	Total Sat. Fat 26.5 grams	3,400 mg Sodium

1450 calorie diet for people < 200 pounds (7 % of diet is 102 calories or   11.3 g of saturated fat)

Time	Food	Calories	Fat	Sodium	Protein
6 AM	Thomas Light Multi-Grain English Muffin	100 calories	1 g fat (0 sat fat)	8 g fiber	
	Velvetta cheese (melt on half muffin)	60 calories	4 g fat (2.5 g saturated fat)	270 mg Na	Protein 5 g
	Simply Jif Peanut Butter (1 Tbsp)	95 calories	8 g fat (3 g sat fat)	65 mg Na	Protein 4 g
	Weight watchers yougurt	100 calories	0.5 g fat (0 sat fat)	110 mg Na	Protein 6 g
	Banana one half on PB	45 calories			
9 AM	Progresso Light Southwestern-style vegetable soup	120 calorie for one can	0 g fat	690 mg Na	Protein 3 g
Noon	Lean Cuisine Chicken Marsala	140 calories	4 g fat (1.5 g sat fat)	620 mg Na	
	Stouffers Beef Pot Roast	240 calories	8 g fat (2.5 g sat fat)	980 mg Na	
3 PM	Hard boiled egg 9 (jumbo size)	100 calories	7 g fat (2 g sat fat)	80 mg Na	Protein 8 g
6 PM	Kashi Black Bean Mango	340 calories	8 g fat (1 g sat fat)	430 mg Na	
	Large salad with Star balsalmic vinegar of Moderna 4 Tbsp	20 calories			
9 PM	Jello Sugar Free Dulce de Leche	60 calories	1 g fat (1 g sat fat)		
	Total calories approx 1450	Total Sat. Fat:	13.5 grams	3,400 mg sodium	

SUPERMARKET SURVIVAL GUIDE: EAT THIS NOT THAT

by David Zinczenko
$13

This book will allow the patient to substitute foods according to taste.

Also the book: *3-Hour Diet* by Jorge Cruise
King Calorie counter for $8

The Skinny on Losing Weight without Being Hungry by Louis J. Aronne, MD, with Alisa Bowman

Some Tubby Diet Pearls

1. If fasting triglycerides are greater than 1,000 mg/dl, restrict total fat to less than 5 g/d to reduce chylomicron triglyceride input. After forty-eight to seventy-two hours, the triglycerides should be less than 1,000.

2. Monounsaturated fatty acids (MUFA) are omega-9s (oleic acid) and have neutral effect on lipids. Sources include olive oil, peanuts, avocados, almonds.

3. Polyunsaturated fatty acids (PUFA) are omega-6s (linoleic acid) and lowers lipids. Sources include flaxseed, soybean and walnuts, canola oil, sunflower oil.

4. Another PUFA are omega-3s (DHA and EPA) which lowers triglycerides and are from oily fish.

5. Another MUFA are trans-fatty acids which raise LDL-C and lower HDL-C but neutral on triglycerides.

6. Stearic acid is a saturated fat from dark chocolate and beef. It is lipid neutral. The problem is fat is 9 calories per gram.

7. The infamous fatty acids are palmitic acid, myristic acid (most potent), lauric acid, and medium-chain fatty acids. They all raise LDL-C.

8. There is 200 mg of cholesterol in the yolk of one egg. That is the daily requirement.

9. The egg is the perfect food as it has all the essential amino acids. Those are the amino acids your body can't make.

My Diet

6:00 am

2 fried eggs (200 calories, 7 g fat [2 g sat fat], 16 g protein)

WeightWatchers yogurt (100 calories, 0.5 g fat, 6 g protein, 110 mg Na)

English muffin

Apple

9:00 am

Atkins Advantage Caramel Double Chocolate Crunch Bar (160 calories, 9 g total fat [6 g sat fat], 160 mg Na, 11 g fiber, 10 g protein)

Noon

Hormel Compleats Spaghetti with meat sauce, ready in 90 seconds (280 calories, 8 g total fat [3.5 g sat fat], 1,300 mg Na, 3 g fiber, 15 g protein)
Progresso Light Savory Vegetable Barley Soup, microwave for 5 minutes (120 calories; 0 total fat; 1,380 mg Na; 8 g fiber; 4 g protein)

3:00 pm

Atkins Advantage Vanilla shakes (150 calories, 9 g total fat [1 g sat fat], 180 mg Na, 2 g dietary fiber, 15 g protein)

6:00 pm

Beef tenderloin 6 oz (402 calories, 24 g fat [6 g sat fat], 102 mg Na, 46 g protein)

Large salad with Newman's Own Lighten Up Balsamic Vinaigrette Dressing 2 tbsp. (45 calories, 4 g total fat [0.5 g sat fat], 470 mg Na)

8:00 pm snack

Orville Redenbachers Smart Pop single serve mini bag (100 calories, 2 g total fat [0.5 g sat fat], 220 mg Na, 4 g fiber, 3 g protein)

Total calories: 2,100 calories

Total sat fat: 20 g

Total protein: 119 g

Total Na: 3,600 mg

Unfortunately, I drink four cups of coffee with 200 calories of cream

I often eat a 12-oz. fillet which adds another 402 calories

I will often imbibe in 10 oz. of red wine 220 calories.

Now I am up to 2,900 calories.

I work out two hours a day, but I still gained 40 of the 80 lb. back.

It is so easy to add up the calories unthinkingly.

Latest Update: *Journal of Clinical Lipidology* (October 2009, volume 3, number 5, page 303-314)

Discussion on Dietary Fat

Clinical Lipidology Roundtable Discussion

Interesting Quotes

Dr. Brown: "There are cross-sectional studies of groups such as Zen Buddhists that suggest that saturated fat intake of around *4%* is a lower limit when consuming natural food substances. It's very hard to go below that number, even on a totally vegetarian diet" (italics mine).

Dr. Rudel: "*Cholesteryl oleate* may be an underappreciated villain" (italics mine).

Dr. Rudel: "*Linolenic acid* doesn't protect against atherosclerosis" (italics mine).

Dr. Rudel: "DHA is not as efficient (as EPA) . . . . they both protect."

Dr. Kris-Etherton: "The clinical and epidemiologic evidence is clear. In a meta-analysis, the 6 trials that studied the replacing of saturated fatty acids with PUFA's reduced the risk for coronary heart disease by 24%.

"Dr. Charles Serhan's work shows that fish oils have marked anti-inflammatory effects by producing the resolvins and protectins"

Dr. Brown: "(Mediterranean diet) is viewed as healthful and as you pointed out the Lyon Diet Heart Study really found that the one fat that correlated best with reduction in events was not monounsaturated *oleic acid*, the major fat of olive oil, it was *linoleic acid*. And so I'm afraid that this has become a great hoax applied to the American diet" (italics mine).

Dr. Rudell: "The polyunsaturated fat diet studies suggests you can lower HDL and still protect, but I think in some cases we can actually do the protection with lower HDL."

Dr. Karmally: "Saturated fat can also increase HDL."

Dr. Rudell: "But this is true for all fat in the diet. The same is true in animals. You know, it's fat in the diet that increases HDL, all kinds of fats do it. Saturated fat does it better than polyunsaturated fat."

My perspective on the above is the following:

1. Everyone needs more fish oil, especially children. Start with DHA/EPA of more than 850 mg a day.
2. Low-fat, low-cholesterol diet lowers LDL-C and lowers HDL-C. The HDL-P is probably the same and still protective.
3. Just eat less calories, and the fat content will take care of itself. Try to eat more protein and less carbs.
4. Find a diet you can stick to the rest of your life, and eat five times a day.

Chapter Twenty-Four

THE TEACHINGS OF THE CHAIRMAN

I passed my lipidology boards in September 2009. My most significant post-lipid board education has come from the Internet blog *Lipidaholics Anonymous Cases* written by *Dr. Thomas Dayspring*.

I will try to summarize the main points to make it more accessible to physicians and perhaps the reading public.

Case 245 (October 25, 2009): Women and CHD: Look Carefully!

> Thus she does not qualify for Framingham risk scoring **(FRS)** and has a low **FRS** of < 10% risk of a CHD event over the next 10 years. Of course the AHA Women's guidelines advises us that any 50 year old woman with a single CHD risk factor has a 50% lifetime chance of a CVD event . . . . So guess what the AHA Women's guidelines state about **FRS**? If the woman scores high, believe it, if she does not score high, **FRS** has little meaning.

I was told by a primary care physician that he decides by gestalt whether a patient is high risk or not. I think that approach misses a lot of high-risk patients. Even using **FRS** misses many high-risk patients. Get a CAC or CIMT to find the high-risk people. This patient had a normal coronary angiogram six years earlier. See what Dr. Dayspring says about this.

> My goodness: a cardiologist who does not know coronary angiograms are simply "*lumenograms*" and that they provide little information about the arterial wall. The angiogram looks at the hole in the middle of the donut not the substance in the fatty, tasty part of the donut (the disease called atherosclerosis) . . . . She had what the card (cardiologist) is calling a false positive stress test: of course he

calls it a false positive because the "lumenogram" (coronary angio) was normal. I'd love to see an IVUS (Intravascular ultrasound) in this woman or a coronary calcium score.

Every physician and patient should understand the above concept. As Glagov stated in the *NEJM* article from 1987, "We conclude that human coronary arteries enlarge in relation to plaque area and that functionally important lumen stenosis may be delayed until the lesion occupies 40 percent of the internal elastic lamina area. The presence of a nearly normal lumen cross-sectional area despite the presence of a large plaque should be taken into account in evaluating atherosclerotic disease with use of coronary angiography." Tim Russert had a normal nuclear stress test one month before he had sudden death. If he had had a repeat CAC or a 128-slice angio or even a CIMT, more would have been known about the cards he had been dealt, that is, his poker hand.

Another point of Dr. Dayspring's to emphasize, "Just published data from NHANES (the National Health and Nutritional Examination Survey) Insulin resistance is likely the most important single cause of CAD. A better understanding of its pathogenesis and how it might be prevented or cured could have a profound effect of CAD.' . . . The reason IR (insulin resistance) is so deadly is through its effect on APOB (LDL-P)" (*Diabetes Care* 2009, 32:361-366).

Insulin resistance, metabolic syndrome are what the Tubby Syndrome is about. Tim Russert had a normal LDL-C of 68. This is not good enough. Get the Tubby *Factor* to less than 80 or better yet get the *APOB* to less than 60 or best of all get the *LDL-P* to less than 750. Then follow the CIMT every two years to make certain you are not getting worse. This is the Tubby plan.

Case 244 (October 4, 2009): LDL-TG vs. LDL-C

Using the NCEP the provider is right this man does not qualify for Framingham Risk Scoring. I for one hope the NCEP dumps or radically improve this outdated way of evaluating risk. It was developed long before we became a very insulin resistant society. Family history, TG, non-HDL-C, APOB are all ignored by FRS.

This is why I love this blog. Dr. Dayspring spells it out beautifully. My reaction in my practice has been to adopt CAC and CIMT as a way to discover subclinical atherosclerosis and treat it aggressively. Primary care physicians don't have the time to do a check-off list to determine risk. These two images will tell us if a patient has plaque. If the patient has plaque, the physician and the patient understand he has a disease that may suddenly kill him.

> We know that the more insulin resistant a patient is, the higher will be the LDL-P.

There are five criteria for metabolic syndrome (Tubby syndrome). The more criteria that are positive, the more insulin resistant the patient is and the more inflammation the patient has.

Case 242 (September 2, 2009): Terrible Lipids, Normal LDL-P (APOB)

This case answers the question, when do LDL-P and APOB miss a diagnosis?
Type III hyperlipoproteinemia.
The incidence of type III is 1/20-30,000 people.
The reason is LDL-P is 90% of the APOB. It does not measure the IDL-P, chylomicrons, and remnants.

The NMR will give the diagnosis of type III as it will show on the second page that IDL-P and VLDL-P are very elevated in the face of a normal LDL-P.

Case 241 (August 20, 2009): Statins and Sterols

> My [Dr. Dayspring's] new approach will be in high and very high risk patients using statins monotherapy (especially high dose), to check absorption/synthesis markers and adjust therapies.

This week, for the first time I ordered *campesterol* and *sitosterol* markers. These are the absorption markers and will identify hyperabsorbers of cholesterol. These are the people who have great responses to Zetia. The hyperabsorbers are the ones who do not respond well to statins.

I have not yet ordered the synthesis markers *lathosterol* and *desmosterol*. Statins decrease production of cholesterol in the liver and lower these two markers of synthesis. The body is in homeostasis and will start absorbing more cholesterol in the gut to compensate. We often notice the LDL-C creep up after time in some patients. These are the patients that should have Zetia added on rather than increasing the statin.

Stellar trial (J. Lipid Res. 2009, 50: 730-739)—Crestor and Lipitor inhibited the marker of synthesis (lathosterol/cholesterol) about the same amount. Crestor increased the marker of absorption (campesterol/cholesterol) by 52% while Lipitor increased the marker of absorption by 72%.

Case 239 (July 23, 2009): Unusual Response to Statin

> The actual tragedy is that > 70% of providers (not doing APOB or LDL-P determinations) do not calculate, enter into the medical record or act upon non-HDL-C.

This is why I have written this book. The Tubby Factor is the non-HDL-C or non-HDL cholesterol. A patient can walk into a doctor's office and ask for the Tubby Factor because he knows that the LDL-C may not be accurate in a patient with the Tubby syndrome. The metabolic syndrome and non-HDL cholesterol do not roll off the tongue as easily as *tubby* does. It is such a great phrase that I have coined I decided to trademark it.

"In the famous Dean Ornish severe fat restriction, angiographic study, plaque disappeared, but the drastic reduction in fat intake reduced both TC and HDL-C. These patients were helped, not hurt by reducing HDL-C."
"Diabetologists may state that unlike NCEP, the ADA Lipid guidelines does have an HDL-C and a TG goal of therapy:(HDL-C > 40 in men, > 50 in women and TG < 150 mg/dl in all).
Dr. Dayspring uses this patient's case to illustrate the absurdity of the ADA's non-evidence based guidelines.

The Tubby guidelines are stricter than the ADA guidelines. I try to raise the HDL-C to 50 in all my patients, and I try to get the TG less than 100. This is why I use Endur-acin 1,000 mg as my second drug after a statin. It lowers the TG and raises the HDL-C and lowers the LDL-C. However I don't keep raising the Endur-acin to raise the HDL to 50. I don't tell patients to drink a glass of wine to get HDL-C to 50. I don't add Trilipex to get HDL-C to 50. Among the forty patients that I have gotten to LDL-P goal less than 750 on statin plus Endur-acin (and sometimes with Zetia as well), twelve patients have HDL-Cs less than 50.

Only one of those is female. Only two patients are less than 40 HDL-C. The ninety-year-old male with a LDL-P of 697 on simvastatin 20 mg, Endur-acin 500 mg BID and Zetia 10 a day has a TG of 234. I am more inclined to increase his fish oil to get this TG down. His HDL-C is 37, and his HDL-P is 29.7. His small HDL-P is 25.6. That is interesting because niacin increases large HDL-P. I don't think this patient needs more medicine.

This is the other "low" HDL-C patient is a seventy-year-old man with LDL-P of 622 on Crestor 5 mg and Endur-acin 500 mg BID. His HDL-C is 33, and his HDL-P is 26.1 with 21.6 small HDL-P. Again a surprise on the small number of large HDL-P in a patient on niacin. His TG is 105. I think I will again follow Dr. Dayspring's advice. If his LDL-P is to goal, the HDL-C and the TG level does not matter. He quotes the NCEP guidelines, "In patients with high TG (between 200 and 500 mg/dl) the NCEP goal of therapy is LDL-C and non-HDL-C [the Tubby Factor]; NCEP would state CASE CLOSED despite the still low HDL-C and high TG." *The patient in this case had a Tubby Factor of 59 and a LDL-C of 16, so NCEP would say case closed despite the TG of 217 and the HDL-C of 24.*

Case 237 (June 24, 2009): Those Misunderstood Triglycerides

Level 1 (empowered randomized double blind, prospective) monotherapy evidence outcomes:

1- Statins: All have solid outcome data
2- Fibrates: Clofibrate and gemfibrozil
3 -Bile Acid Sequestrants: cholestyramine

Drugs with no empowered Level I outcome evidence:

1- Niacin (failed to meet primary outcome data in Coronary Drug Project, which is its only outcome trial)
2- Fenofibrate and Bezafibrate (failed to meet primary endpoint in FIELD and BIP)
3- Ezetimibe
4- Omega-3 fatty acids

How about outcomes with combo products: there is actually only one positive combo outcome trial which few have ever heard of:

Niacin/Fibrate: Stockholm Ischemic Trial. Positive primary and secondary outcomes. Clofibrate and immediated release niacin were used. (Acta Med Scan 1988, 223 [223]:405-418)

This is a great summary that Dr. Dayspring spelled out. We physicians stand on the shoulders of this work.
There are many physicians who do not realize how strong the evidence is. These drugs save lives.

Dr. Dayspring continues with this statement, "So what: we use all sorts of cardiovascular (BP) and diabetes drugs in untested combinations or else we would not achieve BP or A1C goal in many patients."

I can't practice only evidence-based medicine. I use the GISSI and JELIS open-label trials to justify fish oil.
I used the FATS, HATS, and ARBITER trials which are small to justify *niacin* use. The Coronary Drug trial ultimately did show that niacin had decreased mortality after fifteen years. In my judgment this makes statin and niacin the combo therapy of first choice especially because they are available in generic and over the counter.

Dr. Dayspring writes, "Framingham data collected by none other than NCEP chairman Scott Grundy reveals that once non-HDL-C is down, LDL-C is no longer a risk factor for CHD, regardless of a TG above or below 200mg/dl" (2006, *American Journal of Cardiology*, 98:1363-1368).

"For those doing NMR's: APOB consists of VLDL-P + IDL-P + LDL-P

"However, once the the TG are less than 500 mg/dl, non-HDL-C [Tubby Factor] (APOB), not TG becomes the goal of therapy to reduce CVD risk. Look at the patient under discussion. The TG remains high, yet LDL-C and non-HDL-C are at goal, so NCEP would want you to do nothing further despite the TG of > 300 mg/dl . . . . If one wants to be super aggressive (way beyond evidence based medicine) one could make a theoretical case for further reducing the high TG."

Case 235 (May 25, 2009): LDL-C of 7 mg/dl

This patient is on Crestor 5 mg and Niaspan 2,000 mg daily.

His LDL-C is 7 (calculated), and his LDL-P is 716. TG is 308.

Dr. Dayspring writes, "As long as the patient feels well, I certainly would not be too concerned about the LDL-C of 7 per se. The patient has adequate (physiologic) numbers of LDL particles."

He goes on to refer to Dr. Goldstein's article in *Circulation* (2009, 119:2131-2133) that adverse effects such as CNS hemorrhage is not from drug-induced cholesterol reductions.

Also, Dr. Dayspring writes, "Complex hypobetalipoproteinemia (a genetic condition) . . . have LDL-C of 5-20 and most live long and healthy lives without any problem related to cholesterol deficiency."

Case 225 (December 20, 2008): Nobody Dies of High TG

> A TG > 100 is potentially abnormal. Noninsulin resistant populations have fasting TG of 10-70 with a mean of 30. Normal postprandial excursions are 30-100 gm/dl. : thus anyone with a PP (post prandial) TG of > 170 has a pathological condition . . . . If you see a TG of 200 mg/dl do not waste your time asking if the patient was fasting or not: that level is abnormal in either case.

Dr. Dayspring also refers to the Paris Prospective Study which showed CV death associated with TG of more than 133 in diabetic women.

> An LDL and HDL carrying TG is a pathological lipoprotein. Their physiological function is to traffic cholesterol not CE (cholesterol ester), not TG. If you have a lot of LDLs and HDLs carrying TG they contribute to the endothelial dysfunction, coagulation and blood viscosity conditions described above. TG-rich, CE poor HDLs are dysfunctional.

Case 217 (August 24, 2008): Stepping up Particle Biology Knowledge

This is my favorite case. I was lucky enough to be in Cincinnati when he presented this case to a small group including Dr. Allan Sniderman.

The Professor and the Provider

Or are there circumstances where APOB can provide a false negative value. Well, if the immunoassay depends on specific epitopes binding to the antibody (the part of the antibody that binds to the epitope is termed the paratope), what would happen if the configuration of the APOB molecule changed (as could happen when APOB assumes a different configuration on very small LDL particles) or was damaged as might happen when exposed to reactive oxygen species, glycosylation, tyrosination, etc.)

At this meeting, Dr. Sniderman said he was not aware that this occurs.

Chapter Twenty-Five

IF IT AIN'T BROKE, DON'T FIX IT

When I finished my residency in Brooklyn, New York, and moved down to Clermont, Florida, to start a medical practice in internal medicine, I heard for the first time in my life the phrase, "If it ain't broke, don't fix it." Who could argue with that? Yet that is what my practice has evolved into, preventive medicine. I was the fireman in the hospital. I was putting out fires in the intensive care unit. Treating strokes and heart attacks and severe infections, I had patients on ventilators. I heard somewhere that Medicare spends 90% of its funds on the last year of a patient's life. I later did a fellowship in infectious disease. The big issue after HIV was antibiotic resistance. The bugs were smarter than we were. The one area that literally made a disease disappear was vaccination. Preventive medicine. Screening for disease. It used to be that Medicare would not pay for a sigmoidoscopy for screening purposes. Mammograms were also not covered. It is like getting a loan from a bank. You have to have money before they will give you a loan. You need work experience before you can get a job. You can't get the test to find the disease until you have the disease. Eventually mammograms, colonoscopies, and DEX scans were covered by insurance for screening purposes. Presently, CAC CT scans are paid for by Medicare if a patient has a Framingham risk score of 10 to 20%. CIMTs are not covered. I have presented the data of how I used CACs and CIMTs in my practice with NMR LipoProfile. These three tests cost about $400 in my community. Medicare covers NMR LipoProfile. A nuclear stress test costs more than $1,000 with much more radiation exposure. I believe I can prevent my patients from ever needing a nuclear stress test or a coronary angiogram or a coronary bypass. I think I can find the plaque in my patients age 45 and above and then treat for thirty years at less than $100 a year. If it ain't broke, don't fix it. We still need to change the oil in our cars. Let's make sure the pipes in our bodies are kept in as good a shape as we keep our cars.

Chapter Twenty-Five

EVIDENCE-BASED MEDICINE

LEVEL 1: Empowered Randomized Double Blind, Prospective Trials

Simvastatin	4S and HPS
Lipitor	Prove-it
Crestor	JUPITER
Pravastatin	WOSCOPS
Gemfibrozil	Helsinki Heart Study
Cholestyramine	(LRC-CPPT)

Science has proven the above drugs work.

I spoke to a surgeon yesterday who thinks it is all mostly genetics.

That is a travesty. If most of the physicians don't realize the power of the above science, it allows people to continue to look for over-the-counter cures.

A patient told me yesterday that a physician on the radio wasn't convinced about lowering cholesterol. After all, people die with low cholesterols. This was an old problem with the LRC-CPPT study. The cholestyramine group had a 19% reduction in CAD deaths and nonfatal myocardial infarcts ($P < 0.05$). There was no decrease in total mortality. There was an increase (not statistically significant) in noncoronary deaths. A similar problem occurred with the Helsinki Heart Study.

These concerns were addressed in 1995 with WOSCOPS. A 22% reduction in total mortality ($P = 0.051$).

The Scandinavian Simvastatin Survival Study (4S) had an 8% mortality versus 12% with placebo.

The Heart Protection Study had a 13% reduction in all cause mortality.

This question is settled. Lowering LDL-C decreases mortality.

Chapter Twenty-Six

TIMELINE OF IMPORTANT TRIAL STUDIES

In 1913, Professor Anitschow gave rabbits cholesterol.

1961 Framingham Heart Study

1984 CPPT—*The first large double-blinded controlled study* to show reducing cholesterol reduced myocardial infarctions in men with high cholesterol. For seven years, 3,800 men took two packets of cholestyramine three times a day. Cholestyramine causes constipation and is very grainy sludge in liquid. These were an amazing group of patients. Now patients have some muscle pain after lifting something and think it is their statin about to kill them.

1986 Coronary Drug Project Post Hoc Study

Niacin is the first drug to show reduction of total mortality and coronary mortality.

I was in private practice at this time. This was great news. The only problem is I couldn't get anyone to stay on the medicine because of constipation and flushing.

1994 The 4S trial with Zocor

First significant decrease in all-cause mortality. The post hoc study with niacin is not considered "significant" because it did not meet its primary end point back in 1977.

1995 WOSCOPS

First study to show statins safe in patient without having had a heart attack. The decrease in overall mortality was 22%, but it was not statistically significant. It was considered a primary prevention study.

2002 HPS (Heart Protection Study)

Total mortality over 5.4 years was 8% with Zocor.

Total mortality over 5.4 years was 12% with placebo.

The breakthrough CPPT study had an increase in mortality due to suicide.

Total mortality means death from any cause including car accidents, just in case a statin makes you drive poorly.

The CAD deaths had a RRR of 42%. RRR means relative risk reduction. Sounds like almost half the people lived longer, but it doesn't mean that.

Table 7:13 Stone Book
Number Needed To Treat (NNTT)
4S: For all CAD deaths, major CAD event =10
This means you have to treat ten patients to goal before you prevent one CAD death or one CAD event.

NNTT

CARE 33 for all fatal and nonfatal CAD events
VA-HIT 23 for fatal and nonfatal CAD events
WOSCOPS 48 for first fatal and nonfatal CAD events
AFCAPS/TexCAPS 58 for risk of first major CAD event

When you use the NNTT, the statins don't seem so impressive.

I believe we can do much better if we use the LDL-P goal of less than 750 and HDL-C of more than 50 and TG of less than 100.

If we can show regression of atheroma on serial biannual CIMTs, I believe we can virtually eliminate CAD events if we diagnose the vulnerable plaque early with CAC and CIMT.

Find the people who have disease. People have subclinical atherosclerosis if they have no symptoms, but they have a CAC 1.0 or greater or a CIMT more than 25% risk for age.

Goodbye LDL-C

Rest in Peace

In the text *Therapeutic Strategies in Lipid Disorders* by A. M. Tonkin, there is a conclusion from A. D. Sniderman on page 55:

> We do not know in any detail the precise sequence of events that initiates a clinical cardiovascular event and we cannot identify with

any accuracy those who will be the imminent victims. We do know that trapping of an APOB particle within the arterial wall is the cardinal event that initiates and propagates the atherosclerotic process within the arterial wall. We know also that lowering the number of APOB particles within plasma is the single most powerful therapy to reduce injury to the vascular wall and to decrease the number of clinical events . . . . LDL-C and non-HDL-C are imperfect surrogates for APOB. Given that coronary disease is the commonest cause of death worldwide, given that APOB can be measured accurately and inexpensively on non-fasting samples, and given that the superiority of APOB has been acknowledged by the American College of Cardiology, the American Diabetes Association and the American Association of Clinical Chemistry, it is time to introduce APOB into routine clinical practice.

Final Note

Ask your doctor what your Tubby Factor is.

Get a CAC and a CIMT to determine if you are at high risk.

If you are at high risk, get an APOB or an LDL-P level.

"APOB versus Non-HDL-C: What to Do When They Disagree" by Allan Sniderman et al. in *Current Atherosclerosis Reports* (2009, 11:358-363) states the following:

> The battle between APOB and non-HDL cholesterol comes down to a contest between more versus less. Measuring APOB will add more expense up front, but it will also allow more effective diagnosis and therapy because APOB adds clarity and precision to deciding who needs to be treated and how much treatment they require. Therapeutic cost multiples more than tests, and events that are prevented cost multiples less than those that are not. It follows that applying therapies more effectively to those who need them more than others will save more lives and money.

NCEP is making new recommendations. I am hoping they will follow Dr. Sniderman's advice above. However, since I suspect compromise is the essence of committees, I got a trademark on the Tubby Factor.

Let us hope science will win so we can say Tubby Factor RIP.

Afterword

CONFLICT WITH CARDIOLOGISTS

The perception with the public is that cardiologists are specialists in lipidology. Some cardiologists are lipidologists but most are not. After Tim Russert died, none of the cardiologists interviewed discussed the fact that Mr. Russert's non-HDL cholesterol (Tubby Factor) was not at goal.

I recently was referred a sixty-seven-year-old male with an LDL-P of 2,692 and a LDL-C of 189.

Notice the discordance between the two numbers.

LDL-C of 189 is 90th percentile of the population.
LDL-P of 2,692 is 95th percentile of the population.

Under the present NCEP ATP III guidelines, if this patient has only one risk factor (i.e., his age), then drug therapy can be considered for those with LDL-C of more than 190.

This patient has the Tubby syndrome (metabolic syndrome).

He also has asymptomatic PVD and carotid stenosis 9%.

In this poker game of life and death, I wanted to know his CAC (calcium score) and CIMT.

I order a regular treadmill stress test as his FRS was intermediate.

It was a positive stress test.

I thus sent him to the cardiologist to be evaluated as Medicare would not pay for a CAC with a positive stress test.

The cardiologist wrote the following in his consult:

> Dr. Edwards had referred the patient for a carotid intimal study and potentially a coronary calcium score. I do recognize the benefit of those studies in some patients. In this particular case, however, I don't see where we would gain much in terms of decision making . . . I've asked him not to proceed with coronary calcium scoring. If his nuclear perfusion study is abnormal, he will need a cardiac catheterization instead. If his nuclear perfusion study is normal, I have already set his target LDL at less than 70.

The patient had a nuclear perfusion stress test. It was normal.

Tim Russert had a normal nuclear stress test and was at LDL-C goal of 68. He died suddenly one month after his normal stress test.

I wrote the cardiologist that telling the patient he has a normal stress will not motivate him to diet and exercise.

It is a long way from LDL-P of 2,692 to the goal of less than 750 in a very high-risk patient.

This patient will need multiple drugs to get to goal.

He has no symptoms.

He may notice muscle pains when he takes the statin.

His friends tell him statins hurt his liver.

The drugs are expensive, and he doesn't like to take pills.

I need the calcium score number in his brain to motivate him to take his medicine and to diet and exercise.

He still does not know if he has coronary artery disease.

The CAC (calcium score) costs $200, and the radiation exposure is from two to five chest x-rays. The nuclear stress test has much more radiation and more than $1,500.

The CIMT is only $100 and no radiation. We can do it every two years to monitor progression or regression of atheroma.

These are the tools in my tool box to get patients to take medication.

I explained this to another cardiologist, and he said patients usually take his medicine when he orders it.

Not true. Studies show that 70% of patients will not be taking a new perscription when they come back to the office on the next visit.

This is why I wrote the *Tubby Theory from Topeka*. It's been more than a year since Tim Russert's sudden death, and the cardiologist wrote that consult three weeks ago.

The new NCEP guidlelines probably will not make LDL-P, CAC screening, or CIMT screening mandatory.

More than 100,000 sudden deaths outside the hospital each year in the USA.

The public needs to know that we can prevent strokes and heart attacks if we screen for plaque early and to treat LDL-P to goal.

Age	CAC	cimt%	Carotid Stenosis	LDLp	LDLc	Total CHOL	Statin	Endu-racin	Zetia
79	309			653	54	137	S40		Y
79	1500		39	738	31	87	C40	Y	Y
78				728	53	113			
79	+ CATH		9	588	43	98	S40	Y	
78				603	37	115			
83				587	66	145			
82				720	74	154			
83				614	79	169			
83	1700		39	659	74	170	C10	Y	
44				579	79	161			
45				596	61	145			
50		50		681	71	160	S40		
67				741	80	149			
85	0.9		39	594	72	157	C10		
86				740	73	167			
77	+CATH		39	722	8	123	L40	Y	Y
72	11		9	640	60	159	C5		
74				712	50	114			
86				543	56	146	S20		
86	+CATH			586	54	143	C10		
76	+CATH		39	700	32	89	L80	Y	Y
73				679	45	134			
74				541	46	103			
75	+CATH	70	20	469	54	130	S20		
74				474	64	139			
74				471	47	125			
82				505	42	110			
82				670	63	128			
69				624	69	161			
69				451	44	146			
83			POSITIVE	713	58	100	S20		
82				600	73	122			
82				669	77	127			
82				513	57	109			
88				607	52	113			

Age	CAC	cimt%	Carotid Stenosis	LDLp	LDLc	Total CHOL	Statin	Endu-racin	Zetia
88	+		39	591	36	93	S20	Y	
87				561	59	135			
87				739	53	108			
87				519	47	108			
87			39	456	44	109	S40	Y	
55				501	41	119			
55				674	54	132	C5		
92				528	84	173			
93				558	75	172			
93			39	648	64	165			
73				612	84	177			
72				676	53	111			
70				537	47	136			
71	0	<25		732	70	158	P40	Y	
70				493	55	137			
71	+		positive	728	48	129	S80		Y
71				683	38	127			
75				747	35	105			
68	+cath			745	60	162	C10		
54	+cath	50		355	50	278			
69				575	54	96			
69				662	41	98			
70	186	<25		622	43	97	C5	Y	
51				620	58	139			
51				620	58	139	S40		Y
68				631	32	129			
73	43		39	708	51	130			
68				629	83	156			
67				678	61	149			
67	2	<25		605	55	141	C20	Y	
78				684	56	124			
77			9	701	76	147	S40		
77				726	68	144			
76				647	55	138			
67		<25	9	668	72	165			

Age	CAC	cimt%	Carotid Stenosis	LDLp	LDLc	Total CHOL	Statin	Endu-racin	Zetia
67				622	88	184			
81				562	52	120			
80	740			700	42	118	C5		
80				749	48	112			
74	+CATH		59	749	35	127	S40	Y	Y
57		50		686	32	163	C5		
66				460	31	101			
66	+CATH		39	492	37	112	C40	Y	Y
82				484	53	127			
81				608	53	127			
83				456	45	123			
83	11		9	445	52	128	S20		
82				688	60	129			
51				683	51	133			
51	3		9	713	71	171	C5/O		
68				570	54	126			
68				744	63	139			
57	28	50		713	60	127	C5		
84				679	80	171			
52				729	72	151			
63				617	48	102			
69	12		NORMAL	714	68	158	S40	Y	
59	73	>75		639	71	157	C5		
76				607	39	126			
86				586	60	127			
87				566	38	112			
79				606	47	93			
77				666	61	116			
61				725	87	195			
77				667	41	127			
69				511	N/C	166			
88	+		39	694	21	136	S40	Y	
52	3871	<25		401	46	166	C5		
57	0	>75		439	39	138	C10	Y	
69	+cath		9	666	39	100			

Age	CAC	cimt%	Carotid Stenosis	LDLp	LDLc	Total CHOL	Statin	Endu-racin	Zetia
70	+cath		9	748	62	131			
67				516	15	112			
94				660	47	125			
80				694	77	150			
71				744	N/C	131			
74				618	46	100			
75				572	43	98			
90	+CATH		80	697	19	103	S20	Y	Y
60				595	65	137			
77				696	32	112			
83				737	0	105			
80	6	<25		626	29	110	S20		
79				662	38	115			
80				744	41	107			
74				682	58	144			
75	0		9	726	65	157	L40		
74				554	65	165			
63	+CATH		9	555	45	164	S20	Y	Y
68				612	67	142			
77				568	59	118			
78			39	718	46	106	C10	Y	
77				627	59	130			
78				698	52	118			
67				627	27	118			
68				707	35	99			
71				646	48	116			
84				659	66	137			
83				704	63	137			
83				658	56	136			
64				653	60	140			
64	4			714	62	146	S40	Y	
88				577	67	153			
89	+		39	749	63	152	L40	Y	
89				732	59	160			
72	+CATH		9	665	23	124	C20	Y	

Age	CAC	cimt%	Carotid Stenosis	LDLp	LDLc	Total CHOL	Statin	Endu-racin	Zetia
72				656	36	111			
57				730	28	95	C5		Y
71				463	30	106			
69				723	48	107			
69				626	23	105			
69				627	30	108			
76				645	47	107			
87				584	57	119			
56	0		9	681	57	161	C5		
80				523	27	90			
80				705	35	106			
80	+CATH		9	462	27	113	C5		
81				458	55	119			
82				539	71	136			
68				567	46	133			
69				429	44	128			
69	11	50		593	43	129	S10		
70				699	53	127			
43				658	37	64			
55				610	32	93			
54				576	39	105			
55				573	29	103			
55	+CATH			517	33	113	S10		Y
52				696	72	154			
52				667	67	157			
72	+ CATH		POSITIVE	709	65	146	L5/O		
72				706	50	122			
73	20	50	39	678	57	125	C5	Y	
80			9	745	64	161	C10		Y
76				670	74	158			
76				612	67	159			
74				627	53	104			
67				504	80	163			
68				572	63	152			
68	+ CATH		39	294	44	142	L10		Y

Age	CAC	cimt%	Carotid Stenosis	LDLp	LDLc	Total CHOL	Statin	Endu-racin	Zetia
61				706	87	179			
85				405	34	91			
86				712	35	97			
75				737	62	125			
54	1		49	409	84	172		NIA	
74				646	51	128			
75				568	47	131			
74				683	48	138			
85				682	51	111			
86	+CATH		39	734	54	114	S20		Y
85				448	41	110			
71				650	62	136			
70				643	60	145			
55				734	51	120			
68				501	39	103			
69				578	49	105			
69	POS	50		598	53	120	C5	N1000	
76				735	56	140			
72				703	46	93			
72	256		9	592	40	99	S20		
72				513	43	110			
72				716	53	128			
54				669	99	167			
55	0	50		663	72	154			
80				719	44	115			
81				393	38	126			
67				627	59	151			
68	+CATH		39	697	59	148	C10	Y	
67				721	56	142			
62	+CATH		39	695	53	112	S20	Y	
61				718	44	108			
83				676	57	171			
84				560	72	179			
84	33	50		509	65	172	L20	Y	
84				629	75	189			

Age	CAC	cimt%	Carotid Stenosis	LDLp	LDLc	Total CHOL	Statin	Endu-racin	Zetia
48		50		381	39	131	C5		
48				508	39	129			
47				543	57	158			
64	+CATH	>75	9	716	59	153	C20		Y
58				654	36	124			
57				683	33	138			
85				668	41	140			
85	AAA		9	705	41	141	C20		Y
72	1042			679	51	116	L10	Y	
53				724	84	172			
77				700	113	237			
76	5		9	697	71	153	C5		
74				739	80	152			
75			39	645	51	134	S40	Y	
74				707	66	168			
83				354	40	86			
83				706	77	134			
74				605	42	132			
82				622	35	132			
62				743	83	163			
73				602	66	180			
88				605	53	154			
89				520	51	155			
92				527	51	106			
91				506	60	124			
92	374		9	623	52	124	C5/O	Y	
92				600	53	128			
87				674	33	122			
53				741	59	143			
75	PVD		59	574	48	106	L20		
75				732	63	141			
57	+CATH			672	52	106	L20	Niaspan	
87				541	57	112			
83				611	45	117			
83	+CATH		49	637	47	117	L80	Y	

Age	CAC	cimt%	Carotid Stenosis	LDLp	LDLc	Total CHOL	Statin	Endu-racin	Zetia
75				640	55	124			
76	+CATH		39	694	45	126	C40	Y	Y
78				640	30	105			
71	523		59	487	60	165	C10	Y	
70	523		59	691	82	192			
70	523		59	594	72	187			
70	523		59	351	39	160			
82				748	64	131			
82			39	681	56	124	L20		
71				528	28	116			
79	232		39	661	74	161	C5		
79				565	65	145			
79				629	60	148			
74				604	68	158			
82				701	87	210			
84			39	643	45	134	S20		
84				613	52	129			
83				646	73	155			
80				662	76	184			
64				661	55	127			
93				726	36	106			
82			49	737	56	157	C10	Y	
82				688	48	111			
76				725	97	196			
82				730	60	167			
75				723	52	130			
75				707	55	140			
86	+		70	550	56	130			
86				453	38	74			
87				712	66	111			
87				672	56	104			
77				501	65	125			
78				637	56	122			
78	460		9	714	51	124	S20	Y	Y
81				442	69	156			

Age	CAC	cimt%	Carotid Stenosis	LDLp	LDLc	Total CHOL	Statin	Endu-racin	Zetia
82				642	54	122			
81	+cath		39	677	76	190	C5		
77			9	544	52	114			
78			9	734	46	107			
77			9	649	51	117	S40	Y	
89				625	49	146			
89				737	58	166			
91				635	42	109	L20		
84				434	57	143			
84				552	82	167			
84				631	60	146			
85	200		39	660	67	154	S20		
86				516	58	165			
87	+CATH			698	66	170	L40		
86				700	62	176			
87				625	57	174			
88	410		39	607	61	175			
78				480	32	106			
95	104		39	660	50	99	L10	Y	
95				623	48	108			
73				611	48	139			
65	+CATH	50		708	79	156		Y	
72				651	56	145			
71				581	70	150			
88	841		49	690	52	127	C20		
57				677	21	95			
57	100		39	726	51	143			
75	127		49	559	40	113	C20	Y	
84			39	728	51	96			
81				627	56	163			
81			59	736	69	165	PRA40	Y	
75				597	52	113			
75				672	59	123			
54	0	<25		676	46	110	L10	Y	
80				724	69	137			

Age	CAC	cimt%	Carotid Stenosis	LDLp	LDLc	Total CHOL	Statin	Endu-racin	Zetia
69				534	55	117			
69				588	51	113			
67				607	61	134			
67				651	71	137			
68	2751		59	655	61	146	C20	Y	
72				492	43	116			
73			9	363	42	119	S40	Y	
72				670	61	142			
68				703	72	151			
71	+CATH		9	581	59	150	L10	Y	
70				543	69	169			
73				595	61	167			
73				530	30	141			
73			39	588	47	157	S40		
80				652	85	144			
80	0	50		718	93	165	LES80		

Index

LaVergne, TN USA
17 March 2010
176262LV00002B/2/P